Everythi

YOGA

Cover & Graphic Design

Mattias Långström

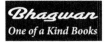

Bhagwan
One of a Kind Books

Everything about YOGA

ISBN 9798838955647

✳ ✳ ✳

2 FREE PREMIUM BONUS!

#1. *Download the **AUDIOBOOK** at the back of the book!*

#2. *Download **CHAKRA-INDEX IN COLOR** here!*
SCAN QR-CODE or go to:
https://bit.ly/47wdFVZ

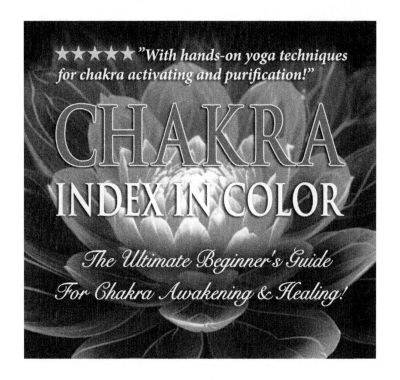

★★★★★ "With hands-on yoga techniques for chakra activating and purification!"

CHAKRA

INDEX IN COLOR

The Ultimate Beginner's Guide For Chakra Awakening & Healing!

FREE PREMIUM Audiobook
Authentic Yoga Nidra Meditation
Integrated Chakra Awakening!

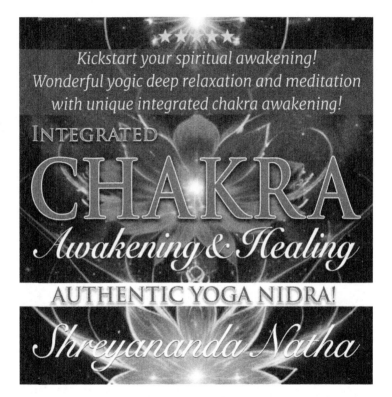

Kickstart your spiritual awakening! Wonderful yogic deep relaxation and meditation with unique integrated chakra awakening!

INTEGRATED

CHAKRA

Awakening & Healing

AUTHENTIC YOGA NIDRA!

Shreyananda Natha

*Download the **AUDIOBOOK** at the back of the book!*

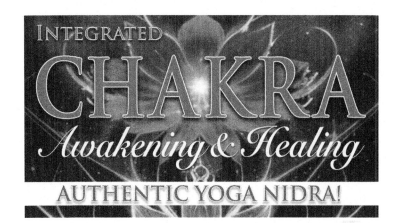

INTEGRATED
CHAKRA
Awakening & Healing
AUTHENTIC YOGA NIDRA!

Kickstart your spiritual awakening! Wonderful yogic deep relaxation and meditation with unique integrated chakra awakening and healing.

PRESENTATION

Yoga Nidra, or yogic sleep, is a unique meditation process that`s powerfully profound and healing for body, mind, and spirit.

Practitioners are led into a state of deep relaxation and the experience of our chakra system.

Yoga Nidra offers extensive benefits, yet it is one of the most straightforward yoga practices.

All you have to do is put on your most comfortable clothes, find a quiet space, lie down on your back, and play the meditation.

Finally, you can read everything about yoga in one book!

Everything About Yoga is the most comprehensive book about yoga, with over 350 pages that are both easy to read and educational. It is an absolute must for future yoga teachers and yoga enthusiasts. Read all about the great yoga paths: HATHA, RAJA, KUNDALINI, KARMA, BHAKTI, JNANA, TANTRA, AYURVEDA & ESOTERIC YOGA (magic mantras, sex magic and yantras).

The book describes – as never before – the great yoga paths, their origins, and their mystery. The book penetrates in depth but remains easy to read, educational, and straightforward. It is a must on the bookshelf for anyone interested in Yoga and eager to know more.

The book covers fundamental yoga philosophy and history topics, including a historical presentation of classical yoga literature: Yoga Sutras of Patanjali, Bhagavad Gita, etc. Each of the significant styles of yoga is described, from Hatha yoga, Raja yoga, Tantra yoga, Bhakti yoga, and Kundalini yoga, to knowledge about the chakras, Ayurveda, and magic mantras, sex magic and yantras.

INCLUDING A PREMIUM AUDIOBOOK: AUTHENTIC YOGA NIDRA MEDITATION – INTEGRATED CHAKRA AWAKE-NING & HEALING!
Kickstart your spiritual awakening! Wonderful yogic deep relaxation and meditation with unique integrated chakra awakening and healing.

Yoga Nidra, or yogic sleep, is a unique meditation process that's powerfully profound and healing for body, mind, and spirit. Practitioners are led into a state of deep relaxation and the experience of our chakra system. Yoga Nidra offers extensive benefits, yet it is one of the most straightforward yoga practices. All you have to do is put on your most comfortable clothes, find a quiet space, lie down on your back, and play the meditation. – **Download the audiobook at the back of the book!**

THE AUTHOR

Shreyananda Natha is the author of popular and best-selling yoga books. He has, among other things, written one of the most comprehensive books about yoga – EVERYTHING ABOUT YOGA and the study book – TEACHING YOGA AND MEDITATION BEYOND THE POSES. He is also a certified yoga and meditation teacher according to the EYTF international guidelines. He has undergone multi-year yoga teacher training under the guidance of Swami Omananda at Satyananda Ashram and holds the highest initiation in the tantric Natha order. He frequently travels to Asia and India to learn and gain knowledge and inspiration. He has immersed himself in tantric rituals and is known for his extensive knowledge of yoga, deep relaxation, and meditation.

"There is no authority that can say what yoga is. When you surrender yourself completely and fully and experience yoga without limitations and doubts, the true encounter with yoga occurs when you become one with the true experience within you. Only then will you understand what yoga is – for you. When you are no longer limited by neatness, shyness, and artificial thought patterns that act as a filter between you and the transformation. Yoga is a cultural-historical wealth still passed on from teacher to student and helps man find his way back to his true nature. It opens us up and attracts awareness. It strengthens our self-esteem, and our person's entire spectrum of possibilities suddenly becomes visible. Yoga is not difficult or strange. You don't have to become a vegan, a monk, or be able to stand on your head. You just need to do your yoga regularly; the rest will take care of itself. You can use yoga and meditation to feel physically and mentally better, achieve success, and develop in all areas of life – here and now. Good luck!"

MY NAME AND MY MISSION

Shreyananda Natha was the name I was given when I was initiated into the Natha Order and received the master mantra – the Shodasi mantra, after studying yoga and tantra for over twelve years, the highest mantra in yoga and tantra. It means "he who knows".

After practicing yoga and meditation continuously for over twenty years, having a yoga school for many years, and leading studies for yoga teachers, I wanted to get out more widely with yoga into our whole society, out of the small yoga room. Spread the knowledge of yoga, our chakra system, and Kundalini Shakti to anyone who will listen. What needed to be added were educational fact books on yoga that didn't just skim the surface or deal with the author's private life. So it became my Sankalpa, my magical wish, and my mission to create exciting yoga books that everyone should be able to read and enjoy. To show how we can apply and use yoga in different areas of life and achieve success and health. Here and now.

If you like my books, feel free to follow me on my social media, share and like, tell your friends about the books, and write an honest review; one or two lines don't matter. All support is precious.

Thanks!

Namasté

I want to thank the teachers and students I've had over the years who have made my journey with yoga so enjoyable. Thank you for all the inspiration you have given me and for making this book possible. The yoga masters who no longer live among us – live on with each new person who immerses themselves in the yoga tradition.

Sri Swami Sivananda, Sri Swami Satyananda, Sri Tirumalai Krishna-macharya, Sri Swami Vishnudevananda, Sri K. Pattabhi Jois, Osho, Swami Nirdosha, Swami Omananda, Swami Janakananda, Ole Schmidt, Turiya, Maryam Abrishami and Sanna Kuittinen.

People who all searched for answers to what they sensed through an activated Ajna chakra. In yoga, they have learned the principles behind the universe, the collective consciousness, and the creative force, Kundalini Shakti. The duality behind everything, both what we see and what we don't see. Together, we are helped to pass on the previously secret knowledge about our gunas, nadis, and chakras to all who want to become a Rishi.

Aum Shri Durgayai Namaha

Shreyananda Natha

INDEX

16

Illuminated

HANDS-ON YOGA TECHNIQUES FOR MANIPURA CHAKRA ACTIVATING AND PURIFICATION

Tanmatra

Jnanendriya

Karmendriya

Tattwa

Bija mantra

Tattwa symbol

Animals

Yoga type

Lotus (Padma)

Anahata

The effects of Anahata in our various bodies:

In annamaya kosha

In pranamaya kosha

In manomaya kosha

Anahata in different stages of gunas

Tamas

Tamas, rajas

Rajas, tamas

Rajas

Rajas, sattwa

Sattwa, rajas

Sattwa

Illuminated

HANDS-ON YOGA TECHNIQUES FOR ANAHATA CHAKRA ACTIVATING AND PURIFICATION

HATHA
YOGA

MY BODY IS MY TEMPEL!

WHAT IS YOGA?

DEFINITION OF YOGA

Yoga chitta vritti nirodha (Yoga Sutras 1.2).
When the mind stills, yoga occurs.

THE MEANING OF YOGA

Yoga means unity and is derived from the word – yuj, which means to
unite in Sanskrit. This unity or connection in the spiritual sense aims
to connect individual consciousness with universal consciousness. In
practice, this aims to balance and find harmony between body, mind,
and emotions—a link between body and soul.

THE PURPOSE OF YOGA

He who knows Kundalini knows yoga. The Kundalini, it's said, is coiled
like a serpent. He who can induce her to move is liberated (Hatha Yoga
Pradipika v.105-111).

The absolute purpose of yoga is to awaken Kundalini Shakti and
make her flow; this is a precondition for human evolution. Kundalini
Shakti flows in the sushumna nadi along the spine and activates our
most important chakras. They are in contact with the brain's untapped
resources. When they are used, latent forces are released, and we are
initiated into the universe's secrets. We become enlightened and get
paranormal abilities – siddhis.

THE GOAL OF YOGA

We can define yoga from a classical perspective, its purpose and
meaning, but there is no authority to prescribe the goal of yoga for

you. Do you want to reach spiritual goals, get help to rid yourself of back problems, or perhaps just be free from demands and stress a few minutes a week?

There is undoubtedly a big difference in the stated goal of yoga if you practice with Aghori sadhus or among orthodox Hindu swamis. Even more significant is the difference between Chinese yoga practitioners and atheists in the Americanized Ashtanga industry. It is and has always been this way; this is the divine essence of yoga. It is as accessible and amorphous in purpose as in the feeling inside us. Yoga is indeed an infinite toolbox. Free to use for what matters most to us. Anandamaya kosha – yoga is unmanifested as our innermost self. When we experience all the power in the universe and on earth – inside and around – we decide for ourselves what the goal of yoga is for us.

THE ORIGIN OF YOGA

The yoga we know today has evolved as part of the Tantric civilization. Some believe the first yogi lived about five thousand years BCE; others believe that yoga is far older than that.

What we do know is that in the Indus Valley in Harappa and Mohenjodaro (Pakistan), where the pre-Vedic people once lived around 2600 BCE, statues depicting Shiva and Shakti (Parvati) have been found through archaeological excavations.

According to the myth, Shiva is the founder of yoga, and Parvati is his first disciple. Shiva is seen as a symbol (embodiment) of the highest consciousness. Parvati is considered the mother of the universe. She is the creator and represents knowledge, will, and action. This power, characterized as Kundalini Shakti, is dormant in every human being.

Parvati conveyed the secret wisdom of human liberation through tantra, where yoga has its roots and cannot be separated, just as consciousness (Shiva) cannot be separated from energy (Shakti).

Yoga originated during the beginning of human civilization. Humans began to discover man's spiritual potential and developed techniques to develop it further. In the past, yoga was kept secret; it was not written down or performed publicly. Yoga was passed on orally from guru to student.

Tantric books are the first to refer to yoga and later to the Vedic scriptures. Rigveda, the oldest Vedic work, was written in 3-5000 BCE, probably by the Indus-Saraswati people. They are a collection of hymns written during a time when the culture in the Indus Valley was flourishing.

According to legend, Shiva (pure consciousness) taught Parvati (Shakti) yoga. A fish overheard their conversation, and Shiva turned the fish into a human. Not only animals would have yoga, but also humans.

VEDIC YOGA / ARCHAIC YOGA
Dating back to 5000 BCE, Vedic yoga is the oldest form. Sacrifice was seen as a path to the union between inner life, the sensual, and outer life, the material. To practice certain rituals and religions based on the Vedic hymns (which can be compared to the Old Testament), one had to focus and concentrate for an extended period, and to achieve this, yogic techniques were developed. Today, this remains the basis of yoga: to use inner focus to increase sensory and human abilities.

Vedic yoga was passed on by rishis (seers), not from guru to student.

PRE-CLASSICAL YOGA

The Upanishads form part of the Vedic scriptures, considered an essential work between 2000 BCE and 200 CE. The Upanishads consist of two hundred Gnostic texts in which yoga is mentioned. Yoga was now taught from guru to student and used to gain insight.

During this time, there were three essential yoga paths:

BHAKTI YOGA *– the path of devotion. It refers to devotion to God or the highest consciousness in any manifestations. A loving relationship with God is developed through acts such as singing and reciting the name of God; this is seen as the easiest path to moksha.*

JNANA YOGA *– the path of knowledge. In Jnana yoga, theorizing gains insight into and understanding the spiritual aspect. Moksha is achieved by understanding that Brahman and Atman are the same.*

KARMA YOGA *– the path of selfless action. The practice of selfless acts unites practitioners with the highest consciousness. You work and help others without taking credit for it. Being fully present in your work makes you a tool for the universe.*

The Bhagavad Gita, seen as a summary of the Upanishads, takes place on the battlefield. Krishna tells Arjuna that he will win the war by following the three yoga paths – Bhakti, Karma, and Jnana yoga.

CLASSICAL YOGA

The critical work for classical yoga (200CE-400CE) was Patanjali's Yoga Sutras – a verse book and one of the six philosophical paths within Hinduism today. Yoga now had its philosophy. Patanjali divi-

ded yoga into eight steps with a focus on concentration. In this context, asanas meant a stable and comfortable position. The physical body was to be steady and immobile during meditation to avoid distraction.

According to Patanjali, an individual comprises Prakriti (matter) and Purusha (soul). Here, the goal of yoga is to stop identifying with the human body, and in doing so, the soul will be liberated and allowed to reunite with the Brahman (universe).

POST-CLASSICAL YOGA

All forms of yoga that came into being after Patanjali are categorized as post-classical yoga (500CE-700CE). Here, tantrism has a significant influence. Unlike in classical yoga, the body and the mind were now seen as one. Previously, the body had been experienced as an obstacle, and meditation was used as a means to the body and worldly matters. This era focused on returning to the origin of yoga: to rejuvenate the body and learn to master it to awaken Kundalini's power. According to tantrism, Kundalini's energy exists in every human being but as a dormant potential; this became the basis of Hatha yoga and the renaissance of tantra. Hatha Yoga Pradipika is an essential work in post-classical yoga.

MODERN / CONTEMPORARY YOGA

Swami Vivekananda (1863-1902) was a Hindu theorist and spiritual leader. He was a student of Sri Ramakrishna and founded the Ramakrishna Mission in 1897. There, they carried out extensive work in healthcare, provided disaster relief, and trained people, among other things. In 1898, Vivekananda attended the World's Fair in the United States, where he introduced Hinduism, which came to play an essential role in the invasion of yoga in the West.

Indra Devi (1899-2001), a German yogi, is another person who played an essential role in the development of yoga. Indra is seen as the First Lady of yoga. At the time, yoga was primarily studied and practiced by men. Indra was active in the yoga industry for sixty years; she taught many different nationalities and has dramatically inspired yogis worldwide. Indra was the first to open a yoga studio in the USA in 1947.

Today's most famous tantric yogi is probably the Dalai Lama.

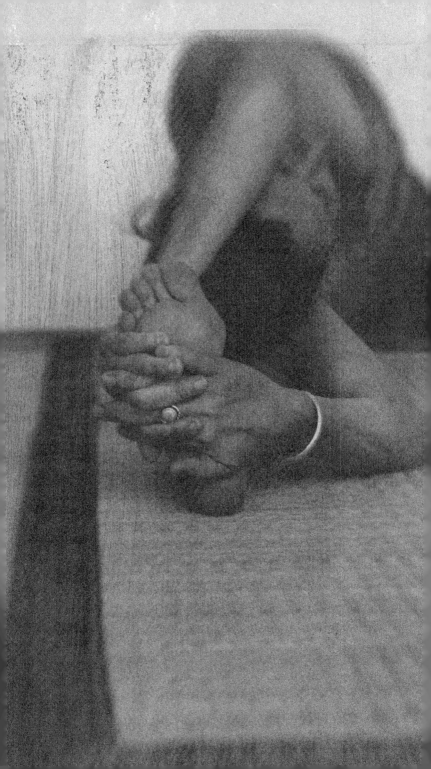

EVOLUTION OF YOGA THROUGH THE 36 TANTRA TATTWAS

36 TANTRA TATTWAS

Man is an image of the universe. The universe is the macrocosm, and man is the microcosm. Everything that is created and that we can see can also be invisible. It comes down to density and goes from the unmanifested to the manifested.

The thirty-six tantra tattwas describe creation from pure consciousness (Shiva) to matter (Shakti); this is represented by thirty-six steps, thirty-six manifestations, of energy that goes from the fine to the rough.

Everything has its beginning in the macrocosm, where there is pure consciousness. There was a densification of consciousness/energy. A vibration was heard – spandam, the sound of Aum, and thus Shakti was manifested.

5 SHIVA TATTWAS
Macrocosm structure

SHIVA

The timeless, eternal space

SHAKTI

The manifested time

ICHA

Will

JNANA

Knowledge

KRIYA

Movement

6 VIDYA TATTWAS

MAYA

Illusion

KALAA

Contraction of KRIYA

VIDYA

Contraction of JNANA

RAGA

Contraction of ICCHA

KALAA

Contraction of Shakti

NIYATI – *contraction* **CHICCHAKTI** *(Shiva)*

25 ATMA TATTWAS
Microcosm; man

PURUSHA   **PRAKRITI**

Shiva   *Shakti*

BUDDHI – *intellect, insight;*
SATTVIC GUNA contr. of JNANA

AHAMKARA – *ego;*
RAJASIC GUNA contraction of ICCHA

MANAS – *thoughts;*
TAMASIC GUNA contraction of KRIYA

5 JNANENDRIYAS
Sound, touch, sight, taste, smell (sense organs, sattvic)

5 KARMENDRIYAS
Speech, feeling, walking, toilet, sneezing (locomotor system, rajasic)

5 TANMANTRA
Sound, taste, shape, smell, touch (sensory attributes, tamasic)

5 MAHA BHUTAS

PRITHVI	APAS	AGNI	VAYU	AKASHA
Soil	Water	Fire	Air	Space

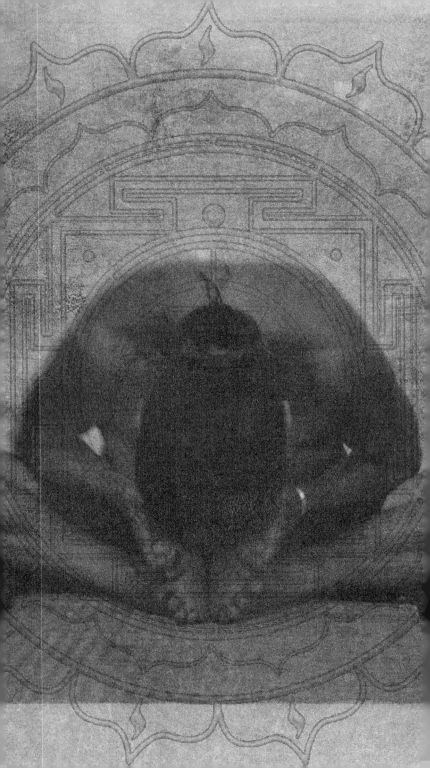

HATHA YOGA

THE YOGA OF BODY CONTROL

Much literature and texts refer to Hatha yoga, most written between 500CE and 1400CE. Hatha Yoga Pradipika by Yogi Swatmarama is one of the most famous. References to Hatha yoga are even made in the Upanishads and Puranas, written long before Buddhism (about 500 BCE). Traces of Hatha yoga have also been found in pre-Columbian culture in America. Even today, giant stone figures in St. Augustine in South America represent Hatha yoga asanas.

Hatha yoga is associated with Gorakhnath, a leading guru in Hatha yoga (approx. 500 CE-1100 CE). Gorakhnath was a disciple of Matsyendranatha, the first guru in Hatha yoga. Matsya means fish.

Buddha and Mahavir, the founders of the Jain sect, were two important figures in India around 500 BCE. At that time, man's spiritual development had been ongoing for centuries.

Two of the Buddha's teachings became known worldwide: Vipassana and Anapanasati. For these, the Buddha created a system called the Eightfold Path. This system deals with ethics and correct livelihood and has remarkable similarities to Raja Yoga's yamas and niyamas. Meditation became a popular method of spiritual development. However, they had no preparatory steps for meditation and eventually began to try the Buddha's system. Meditation was considered the highest path, but it was acknowledged that some preparations were required before practitioners could meditate.

Five hundred years after the time of the Buddha, a Buddhist university was established in Nalanda, Bihar, India. It was called the Hinayana system and was an orthodox Buddhist system.

At the same time, another university was established in Vikram Shila, Bihar, India. It became a learning center espousing the Mahayana tradition. They disagreed with the orthodox interpretation of the Buddha's teachings, viewing the Hinayana system as a deviation from the Buddha's teachings. The Mahayana tradition was founded by a group of liberal Buddhists who now began to embrace tantric thinking and philosophy.

After the fall of Buddhism in India (300 CE-500 CE), some great yogis wanted to return to the original doctrine of yoga and tantrism. Matsyendranatha and Goraknatha were two of these. They thought the essence of the principle had been forgotten and misunderstood by many. They separated Hatha and Raja yoga from the tantric rituals and developed the most useful, practical exercises in yoga and the tantric system. It also became necessary to reintroduce a proper meditation system. In this way, Hatha yoga was established. Matsyendranatha founded the Natha order.

To cleanse the body and its elements before meditation is the foundation of Hatha yoga. In Hatha yoga, body and mind are seen as one and equally important.

THE FIVE ELEMENTS OF HATHA YOGA:

ASANAS
In Raja yoga, asanas refer to a comfortable and steady position. Hatha

yoga asanas are specific postures that help open our energy channels and centers. Hatha yogis discovered they also gained control over the mind through reasonable body control. Therefore, asanas are put at the forefront of Hatha yoga.

PRANAYAMAS

Breathing influences the flow of prana in our nadis (energy channels). Breathwork is a method through which breathing exercises activate, regulate, and purify our life energy in the energy body. You get a higher degree of power and increase your consciousness.

MUDRAS

Mudra can be translated as posture or gesture. Various energy points are stimulated through mudras, affecting our body and mind. Mudras can influence your mood and deepen your concentration and consciousness. You hold on to and redirect prana through mudras, which would otherwise disappear from the body. In this way, mudras also play an important role in awakening Kundalini Shakti.

BANDHAS

Traditionally, bandhas are classified as part of mudras. Bandhas are often combined with mudras and pranayamas, but they are an essential group of exercises in their own right. Bandha means lock, which describes movement and its effect on our energy body. Prana is locked in specific areas of the body, and the flow of prana to the sushumna nadi is controlled, which develops our spiritual awakening.

SHATKARMAS

Shatkarmas are a series of purification processes divided into six groups. These aim to create harmony between ida and pingala nadi to achieve mental and physical balance and purity. Purification processes are also used before breathing exercises to expel toxins from the body.

HATHA YOGA PRADIPIKA

Hatha Yoga Pradipika is a classic textbook on Hatha yoga. It was written in the fifteenth century by Swami Svatmarama, a Swami Gorakhnath disciple. Hatha Yoga Pradipika is thus the oldest preserved Hatha yoga text and one of the three classical texts, next to Gheranda Samhita and Shiva Samhita.

The book contains a total of three hundred and ninety verses. Of these, about forty are dedicated to asanas, about one hundred to pranayamas, one-hundred-and-fifty to mudras, bandhas, and shatkarmas, and the rest to pratyahara, dharana, dhyana and samadhi. The book consists of four chapters:

1.) Asana: Svatmarama honors his teachers and explains why he wrote the book and who he wrote it for. He describes how and where yoga should be practiced. Svatmarama then describes fifteen asanas and gives recommendations for eating habits.

2.) Pranayama: Svatmarama addresses the connections between breathing, mind, Kundalini, bandha, nadi, and prana. He then describes six karmas and eight kumbhakas.

3.) Mudras: The author describes ten different mudras.

4.) Samadhi: Svatmarama discusses samadhi, laya, nada, two mudras, and the four steps of yoga.

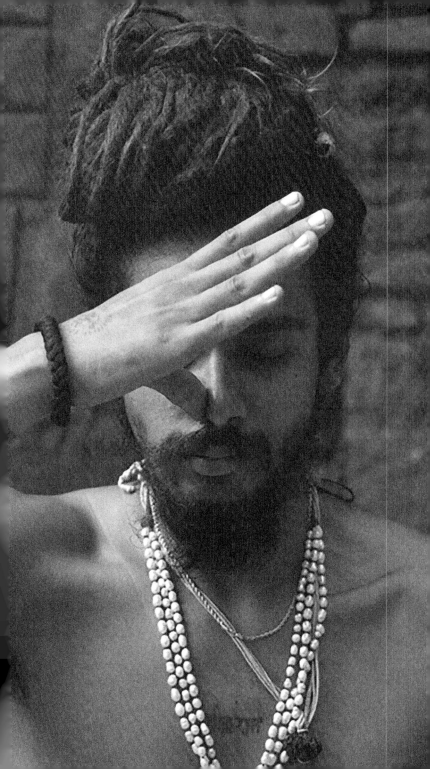

Hatha Yoga Pradipika is dedicated to Lord Adinatha, another name for Shiva (a Hindu god of destruction and renewal), and is believed to have revealed the mysteries of Hatha yoga to his divine consort Parvati.

HE WHO KNOWS KUNDALINI, KNOWS YOGA

THE KUNDALINI, IT'S SAID, IS COILED LIKE A SERPENT

HE WHO CAN INDUCE HER TO MOVE IS LIBERATED

(Hatha Yoga Pradipika v.105-111)

ADVANCED HATHA YOGA

OUR FIVE SHEATHS

Our physical body, the three bodies of the astral body, and our inner-most interior.

Hatha yoga teaches that we consist of five sheaths or bodies:

ANNAMAYA KOSHA

Physical body.

PRANAMAYA KOSHA

Energy body.

MANOMAYA KOSHA

Mental body.

VIGYANAMAYA KOSHA

Wisdom Body.

ANANDAMAYA KOSHA

Bliss body (pure consciousness of true self).

The energy body, the mental body, and the wisdom body form the astral body.

NADIS – IDA AND PINGALA AND SUSHUMNA NADI

Pranamaya kosha – our energy body – consists of about seventy-two thousand nadis (subtle channels through which prana flows). It is the energy body that gives us life. The three most important nadis are ida,

*pingala, and sushumna nadi, of which sushumna nadi is the most
important.*

*Ida nadi flows from the left side of the spine and controls mental energy. It is associated with the parasympathetic nervous system. Pingala
nadi flows along the right side of the divide and controls our physical
body. It is associated with the sympathetic nervous system. Sushumna
nadi, the most important of the three, flows along the entire spine and
channels the spiritual energy.*

*Ida and pingala nadi flow from the root chakra and cross the sushumna nadi at four places in the body to finally unite at the eyebrow
center. Ida nadi then goes out through the left nostril and pingala nadi
through the right.*

*We can regulate the body's energies through asanas, and when ida and
pingala nadi flow simultaneously, sushumna nadi opens. Kundalini
Shakti can begin to travel upwards and activate our chakra system,
illuminating our brain's dormant parts. Usually, we use about twenty
percent of our brain capacity. Special siddhis, paranormal abilities,
arise on our path to activating a more significant part of the brain. You
become a Siddha. However, these abilities are not the ultimate goal.*

HA + THA
*Ha – pingala nadi – the sun stands for the sympathetic nervous system,
and tha – ida nadi – the moon stands for the parasympathetic nervous
system.*

OUR SUBTLE ENERGY BODY WITH FIVE PRANA VAYUS
Our five bodies interact with each other and create a whole. The

breathing exercises mainly affect our energy body – pranamaya kosha,
which comprises five different types of sub-pranas. These five prana
vayus (wind) are prana, apana, samana, udana and vyana. The link
also binds the bodies together and affects us in all directions. If we
calm the body with breathing, we also calm the mind and vice versa,
which you probably have experienced during your yoga practice.

PRANA

In this context, prana does not refer to the cosmic prana but to the
flow of energy that controls the thorax area between the larynx and
the diaphragm. This area is linked to the heart and respiratory system,
along with the muscles and nerves that activate them. It is this power
that makes us draw inward breath.

APANA

Apana controls the abdomen and the area under the navel, providing
energy to the intestines, kidneys, rectum, and genitals. It affects the
expulsion of waste products in the body and is the force that makes us
exhale.

SAMANA

Samana is located between the heart and the navel. It activates and
controls the digestive system. Samana is responsible for the transfor-
mation; physically, the transformation refers to the very distribution of
nutrients in the body, and evolutionarily, it relates to Kundalini power
and the development of our consciousness.

UDANA

Udana controls the area of the neck and head. It activates all our sen-
sory receptors, including eyes, tongue, nose, and ears. Udana activates

and balances muscles, ligaments, nerves, and joints in our arms and legs. It is responsible for our posture, sensory attention, and ability to interact with the outside world.

VYANA

Vyana permeates the whole body. It regulates and controls all our movements and coordinates all sub-pranas in the body.

In addition to the most critical sub-pranas, five smaller pranas are called upa-pranas. These five are naga, koorma, krikara, devadatta, and dhananjaya. Naga is responsible for belching and hiccups; koorma opens our eyes and makes us blink; krikara creates hunger, thirst, sneezing, and coughing; devadatta generates sleep and yawn; and dhananjaya activates when we die, and our body begins to break down.

PRANA AND LIFESTYLE

Our lifestyle has a significant impact on our energy body and its prana. Physical activity such as exercise, work, sleep, food, and sexual relationships affect the distribution and flow of prana in our body. Emotions, thoughts, and fantasies affect our bodies even more. An unbalanced lifestyle, poor diet, and stress break down and block the flow of prana. It results in feeling drained of energy. When energy becomes low in one of our sub-pranas, the very area of the body that the prana controls is affected and may result in illness. Breathing exercises can prevent this by balancing or increasing the energy in our energy body.

ASANA

There is a definition of asanas – Stirham Sukham Asana – in Patanjali's Yoga Sutras, which means steady or comfortable position. They wanted to develop their ability to sit still for a long time because it was a prerequisite for meditation.

In Hatha yoga, however, it was discovered that specific postures, asanas, opened up energy channels and mental centers in the body. You have better body control and could thus also develop control over the mind, thoughts, and energies. Yoga asanas became a tool for achieving higher consciousness and provided a stable foundation to explore the body, mind, and breathing.

Initially, there were eight-million-four-hundred-thousand different asanas. These represent as many lives an unenlightened person must be reborn into before becoming enlightened. Rishis and yogis scaled down the number to the few hundred known today. Of these, the eighty-four most important asanas were then highlighted. Thirty-five asanas have a direct impact on our chakras. The others purify and regulate our nadis. Asanas create a balance between body and mind and a flow in the sushumna.

Rishis studied the animals and noticed how they lived harmoniously with their bodies and surroundings. By mimicking the animals' movements and postures, hormone secretion in the body was affected. During deep meditation, they observed how different poses affected the body and the mind.

Prana, the vital energy (life energy), permeates our entire body—a poor flow of prana in the body results in stiffness and an accumulation of toxins. When prana flows freely, these toxins are removed, and the body becomes soft and supple. Even the most challenging postures are easy to perform because when the amount of prana increases in the body, pranic intuition is achieved. An intuitive sense of how to perform asanas, mudras, and pranayamas follows.

Hatha yoga increases overall health and activates our energy centers by balancing the nervous system.

Asanas in Hatha yoga release tensions that arise as knots in our muscles. By removing these tensions from the body, we also release tensions from the mind. It makes us feel better in general and releases underlying and hidden energy that lies latent.

Thus, asanas are more than exercise. They are techniques that place the body in different positions to promote awareness, relaxation, concentration, and meditation. Part of this process is to develop a good physique through stretching, stimulation of prana, and massage of the glands and internal organs.

Asanas are divided into three groups: beginners, intermediate and advanced. It is optional to complete all the exercises in each group. Daily practice of a tailor-made program will have the most significant effect.

Those who have never practiced yoga should perform asanas for beginners. These have a more significant effect on beginners' bodies than advanced exercises. These exercises prepare the body and mind for more advanced exercises and meditation and help improve physical health.

The intermediate asanas are for those who can efficiently complete the exercises for beginners. These require greater concentration, steadiness, and coordination with movement and breathing.

Advanced asanas are for those with well-developed body control, muscles, and nervous system. You should be able to master the intermediate exercises without problem. It is essential to take your time and start these exercises early enough.

DYNAMIC AND STATIC ASANAS

*Dynamic asanas increase flexibility and circulation in the body.
They soften muscles, release knots and energy blockages, and remove
stagnant blood. These asanas are most important for the beginner. To
start work with the chakra system, for example, blockages must first be
released; otherwise, the energy may flow the wrong way in the energy
body. Dynamic asanas and vinyasa process our physical body; they
take us deeper and prepare us for the more static asanas. Hatha yoga
often starts with a lot of movement and gradually lets the vibrations
subside into stillness and silence. It has much to do with moving from
the rough to the fine – from the body to the mind – and knowing how
yoga affects our doshas through Ayurveda.*

VINYASA

*Dynamic asanas are often synchronized with breathing. When we
do that, it's called vinyasa—a flow where movements and breathing
interact.*

*Vinyasa aims to increase the internal cleansing and detoxification of
the body. Breathing synchronized with movement warms the blood.
Thick blood is often unhealthy and causes diseases. The heat from vinyasa cleanses the blood and makes it thinner so it can circulate better in
the body and around our joints, reducing pain.*

*Where there is poor circulation in the body, pain usually occurs. The
heated blood also passes through all the internal organs. It transports
impurities and diseases removed from the body with our increased
amount of sweat during the yoga session.*

Sweat is an essential by-product of vinyasa. It is only through our sweat that diseases can leave the body and be purified, in the same way, that gold is melted to eliminate its impurities. Yoga boils the blood and transports contaminants and toxins to the surface, which are then removed with the help of sweat. If you practice vinyasa often, the body becomes healthy, strong, clean, and shiny like gold.

With the body cleansed, it is possible to cleanse the nervous system and sense organs.

STATIC ASANAS

Static and, above all, inverted asanas have the most profound effect on our energy body and our chakra system. These require greater flexibility and are suited for more experienced practitioners. Remaining in the position for a few minutes has a more powerful effect on the glands, prana, chakras, and internal organs. The mind becomes calm and prepares the individual for meditation. Some static asanas are beneficial for reaching pratyahara.

TRISTHANA

Tristhana means three areas to pay attention to: postures (position, stretching, and relaxation), breath, and gazing point. They are always performed in conjunction with each other.

Asanas cleanse, strengthen, and soften the body. We cleanse the nervous system when we breathe with rechaka and puraka, a steady and even inhalation and exhalation at the same pace. Drishti is the place you look at during yoga practice. There are nine different ones: the tip of the nose, eyebrow center, navel, thumbs, hands, feet, right and left side, up to the sky. Drishi purifies, captures, and stabilizes the mind.

ADVICE FOR THE PRACTICE OF ASANAS:

BREATH

According to Hatha yoga, two components are needed to cleanse the body internally: the elements air and fire. Fire, our life force, is located at the solar plexus in the body and is generated by the Manipura chakra. Air is required for fire to burn, hence the importance of proper breathing in yoga. Long, even breaths increase the internal fire in the body, which heats the blood for physical purification and burns up impurities in the nervous system. As the inner fire increases in strength, so does our digestive system, health, and longevity. Uneven breathing creates an imbalance in our physical body and its signaling system, weakening our immune system. We risk becoming ill in the long run – according to Hatha yoga, we tolerate stress and toxins less.

Another critical component to increase the inner fire is moola and uddiyana bandha: root and stomach locks. They increase the effect of breathing, keep it inside the body longer, encapsulate the energy, and provide light, strength, and health to the body. According to Hatha yoga, six toxins in the body surround our spiritual heart. The light in our heart is obscured by these six poisons: kama, krodha, moha, lobha, matsarya, and mada. They are desire, anger, delusion, greed, envy and sloth. When we practice Hatha yoga for an extended period with power, determination, and proper breathing, the increasing heat in the body will burn up these six toxins, and the light in our interior will shine through.

Breathing through the nose (unless otherwise stated) and coordinating breathing with movement is essential. But never force yourself to breathe through your nose. If you need to breathe through your mouth,

*do it. Your fine energy channels can be damaged otherwise, and the
energy will flow the wrong way in the energy body. If you are panting,
wait until you can breathe through your nose again more quickly.*

CONSCIOUSNESS
*The purpose of asanas is to influence and create harmony in all aspects
of man: physical, mental, emotional, pranic, and spiritual. By performing asanas consciously, all these parts are affected. One should be
aware of body sensations, movement, and posture on its own and in
coordination with breathing, the flow of prana, focus on the chakra
and witness thoughts and feelings that come up.*

RELAXATION
*You can lie down in shavasana at any time for rest or contemplation.
Notice how it feels in the body.*

SERIES
*You always begin with shatkarmas (purification processes), such as
nasal rinsing (jala neti). Then you perform asanas, pranayamas,
pratyahara, and dharana (concentration / quiet the mind), leading
to dhyana (meditation). You can also add both breathing exercises
and meditation before asanas. It fulfills a function – especially at the
beginning of your yoga practice that you go from the outside in (see
the text about our five bodies) before you intuitively know what, when,
and how to do it.*

OPPOSITION
*It is essential to have a structure in the program to balance the body
and nervous system. A backward bending and vice versa should always
follow a forward bending position. However, this does not apply to
yoga rehabilitation.*

TIME

Asanas can be practiced at any time of the day, provided you have not eaten a few hours prior. That said, practicing just before sunrise and sunset is recommended. The time of day just before daylight is called Brahma muhurta (the divine time – God's time). The atmosphere is still clean, the stomach and intestines inactive, and the mind still. The most favorable time is before sunrise and sunset, but do not be too ambitious. A yoga session during the day is better than having no session.

PLACE

One should find a secluded place that is tidy, clean, quiet, and peaceful. No furniture or objects should be in the way. You can also practice outdoors in a comfortable and beautiful place, not in the cold and wind, where the air is unclean, or in the scorching sun.

CHOICE OF YOGA MAT

Use a mat made of natural materials. It has the most beneficial effect on our pranic currents. Choose a yoga mat you can use for many years to come of the best quality; the prana is stored in the mat and has a beneficial effect on the body. So, take care of your yoga mat and treat it tenderly. Make sure that you can lie on it comfortably and that it is not too small or too thin so that the surface is felt if you, e.g., standing on the head. It should be damping but, at the same time, provide a good grip. A good yoga mat will last at least ten years or longer, so don't be stingy with yourself. Treat yourself to a premium yoga mat of the right size and with the right feeling.

CLOTHES

Wear loose and comfortable clothes, remove jewelry, and be barefoot so you do not slip.

SHOWER

Try to take a cold shower before the session to wake the body up. After the session, wait to shower so you do not unnecessarily cool down your body too quickly and lose the healing effect of yoga.

LOO

Empty the stomach.

DIET

There are no strict rules regulating what food to eat. However, a natural diet in moderate amounts is recommended so that not all energy is used to digest food. A vegetarian diet is not essential, but it is recommended. The stomach should be filled half with food, a quarter with water, and a quarter should be left empty. However, do not drink water during the practice as it draws blood and energy to the stomach and cools down your energy body. Also, wait two to three hours to practice yoga after eating so it does not feel uncomfortable during the session.

PERFORMANCE

Asanas are performed softly and gently in three steps:

Awareness of the body, movement, and thoughts creates calm, balance, and focus, leading to a state of harmony in the body.

Awareness of breathing. Synchronize movement with breathing. The action becomes calmer, and brain waves become slower. You become relaxed and gain an increased understanding.

Awareness of the flow of prana can be experienced as tingles in the body. The feeling is developed through regular practice. You become mentally calm, focused, and emotionally receptive.

Asanas are also divided into three parts:

Starting poses.
Implementation.
Final poses.

IMPORTANT
A physician should be consulted before performing asanas in the event of any injury or illness.

Asanas must never hurt joints, complex parts, or ligaments during practice.

Inverted asanas should be avoided during gas formation (toxins can reach the brain), late pregnancy, and menstruation (the cycle can be disrupted). Never sunbathe immediately following yoga practice to avoid overheating.

PRANAYAMAS
Pranayama means breathing technique or breathing control and originates from the words prana – (life force or life energy), yama (discipline or power), and ayama (extension, restraint, or expansion). Pranayamas are divided into puraka (inhalation), kumbhaka (retention of breath), and rechaka (exhalation). Kumbhaka, in turn, is divided into bahir (the retention of breath immediately following exhalation) and antar (holding your breath inside after inhaling). In yogic writings, kevala kumbhaka is also mentioned. It is an advanced yogic condition where breathing via the lungs stops spontaneously, and energy (prana) seeps through the pores in the body's cells.

HEALTH AND BREATHING

Breathing is the most important function we have in the body. It affects the activity of every single cell, including the brain and its operations. A person breathes about fifteen breaths per minute and about twenty-thousand-six hundred breaths daily. Most live incompletely, using only a tiny part of our lungs' capacity. The breathing then becomes shallow, and the body becomes poor in oxygen and prana, which are necessary to maintain good health.

Rhythmic, deep, and slow breathing encourages and is encouraged by a calm and satisfied state of mind. Irregular and uneven breathing disrupts the brain's rhythm, leading to physical, emotional, and mental blockages. It, in turn, causes internal conflicts, an unbalanced personality, a disordered lifestyle, and illness. You build a regular breathing pattern and break this vicious circle through breathing exercises. We learn to regain control of breathing and rebuild our body and mind's natural, relaxed rhythm.

Despite being an unconscious process, you can turn breathing into a conscious process at any time; it creates a link between the unconscious and conscious parts of our mind. The energy that is absorbed by neurotic and unconscious mental patterns can be released with the help of breathing exercises. The energy can then be used on something creative and joyful.

BREATHING AND LIFE

Ancient yogis and rishis studied nature in detail. They noted that animals with slow breathing had a long lifespan, and animals with fast breathing only lived for a few years. Through this observation, they realized how crucial slow breathing is for longevity. Physically, breathing

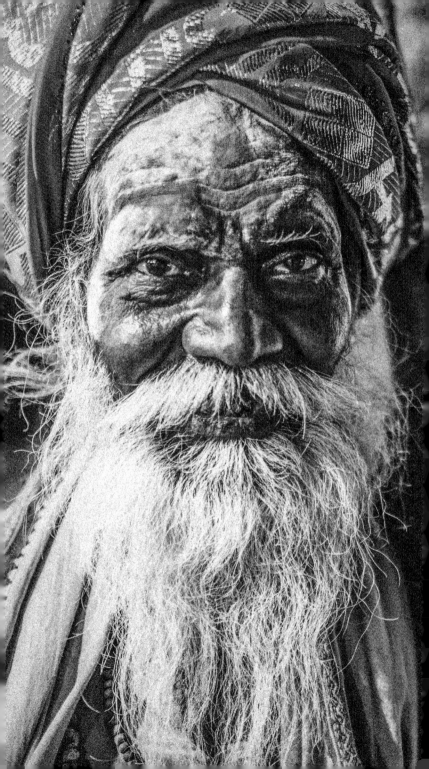

is directly linked to the heart. Slow breathing keeps the heart strong, which leads to a longer life. Deep breathing also increases the absorption of energy in our energy body, which increases mobility, vitality, and well-being.

BREATHING EXERCISES AND THE SPIRITUAL SEARCH
Breathing exercises build a healthy body by releasing blockages in the energy body, increasing the absorption and retention of prana. A calm and quiet mind is a prerequisite for spiritual exercises. In many breathing exercises, kumbhaka (retention of breath) controls the flow of prana, calms the mind, and controls the thought process. When the mind is calmed down, and prana can flow freely through our nadis and chakras, the development of our consciousness is enabled; it, in turn, can lead us to higher dimensions of spiritual experiences.

COMMON ADVICE
Contraindications. Breathing exercises should not be practiced during illness. However, lighter exercises such as conscious or abdominal breathing in shavasana are still acceptable.

TIME
The best time for breathing exercises is in the morning before sunrise. The body is calm, and the mind is still, as it has not yet had time to absorb many impressions from its surroundings. If this is impossible, the second-best time is in the evening when the sun goes down. Soothing breathing exercises are good to do before falling asleep. Try breathing exercises simultaneously and in the same place every day. Regular practice builds strength and willpower.

HYGIENE

Take a bath or shower before practicing pranayamas. At least wash your hands, face, and feet. Please wait at least half an hour to bathe after completing breathing exercises; it is to allow the body temperature to normalize.

FOOD

Eat your breakfast after completing the practice, or wait three to four hours after eating to practice. With food in the stomach, pressure forms on the diaphragm and lungs, making breathing difficult to deeply and completely. It hinders the use of the total capacity of the lungs.

When you start practicing breathing exercises, you may experience constipation and a decrease in urine. If this occurs, reduce salt and spices, and drink plenty of water. Should you encounter an anxious stomach and an increase in urine, take a break from practice for a few days.

PLACE

Practice in a place where you can find peace and where it is clean. The area should be well-ventilated, but not so you are sitting in a draft. Avoid direct sunlight as it may cause overheating.

BREATH

Always breathe through your nose unless otherwise instructed. The air must be able to flow freely through both nostrils.

SEQUENCE

Breathing exercises are done after shatkarmas, often after asanas, and before meditation, but can also be practiced before asanas. Nadi

shodana should be included in each breathing exercise. Lie down in
shavasana for a few minutes after completing the asanas.

SITTING POSITION

A comfortable sitting position is necessary to keep the body and bre-
athing stable during the exercises. The body should be as relaxed as
possible with a straight spine and neck. The mat should be made of na-
tural material. If you cannot sit comfortably in a meditation position
for a long time, you can sit against a wall with outstretched legs or on a
chair with a straight backrest.

Avoid exertion. It is important to remember not to exert too much
effort when doing breathing exercises. Take your time to advance.
Only move on to the next step once you feel entirely comfortable with
a routine. Keeping your breath inside/out is only achieved as long as it
feels comfortable.

SIDE EFFECTS

Various physical and mental symptoms can occur in normally healthy
people. Physical symptoms occur as a result of the detoxification of
toxins. Feelings like tingling, heat and cold, lightness, and heaviness
may occur. These are usually temporary. Energy levels may increase or
fluctuate, and interests may change. If these changes create problems,
you should seek the guidance of a competent guru. Excessive pranaya-
mas late at night can lead to sleeping problems and an extreme excess
of energy the next day – what many wrongly describe as a Kundalini
awakening or hypersensitivity. Pranayamas are powerful tools and
should be treated with respect. Slightly simplified, you can say that
through breathing exercises, agni (fire) is increased in us, and Ma-
nipura chakra at the navel increases its activity; it causes vayu (air)

attached to the chakra above, Anahata, to be netted and expanded. As
the air expands, so does the space within us (Akasha), and a more profound spiritual experience is reached. However, increasing the amount
of vayu can lead to anxiety and worry, so you must end each session by
reducing the excess of vata you have built up. Excessive practice can, in
the worst case, lead to psychosis and delusions.

MUDRA / GESTURE

Mudra can be translated as posture or gesture. Various energy points
that affect both body and mind are stimulated through mudras. Your
mood is influenced, and your consciousness and ability to concentrate
are increased. With the help of mudras, you can hold and control prana that would otherwise disappear from the body. Hence, mudras also
play an important role in awakening Kundalini's energy. Mudras can
be done as a single exercise or in combination with asanas, pranayamas, bandhas, and different visualization techniques.

In Hatha Yoga Pradipika, mudras are discussed as "yoganaga": a separate branch of yoga that requires a subtle presence. You often learn these techniques after you have become accustomed to and knowledgeable
in asanas, pranayamas, and bandhas and when you have eliminated
blockages from the body. Mudras are among the more advanced techniques that awaken our prana, chakras, and Kundalini Shakti, which
can open up various siddhis (paranormal or mental forces) in the more
advanced practitioners.

Mudras create a direct link between annamaya kosha (our physical
body), manomaya kosha (our mental body), and pranamaya kosha
(our energy body); it increases the feeling and awareness of the flow of
prana in the body. A pranic balance is created in our koshas, and the

subtle energy is directed to the higher chakras, promoting increased consciousness.

Our nadis and chakras radiate energy, which usually disappears from the body into our surroundings. By creating barriers within the body with the help of mudras, the energy is instead directed inwards. According to Tantric literature, when prana is kept in the body with the assistance of mudras, the mind becomes introverted, which leads to pratyahara – withdrawal of our senses – as well as dharana (concentration).

Mudras can be divided into five different categories:

HASTA / HAND MUDRA

These lead the energy created in our hands back into the body. You create an energy path that flows from the brain to the hands and back again. If you know this process, an inner awareness is completed quickly. Mudras in this category are: jnana mudra, chin mudra, yoni mudra, bhairava mudra, and hridayamudra.

MANA / HEAD MUDRA

These techniques are essential to Kundalini yoga; many are meditation techniques. Here, you use eyes, ears, nose, tongue and lips. Mudras in this category are: shambhavi mudra, nasikagra drishti, khechari mudra, khaki mudra, bhujangini mudra, bhoochari mudra, akashi mudra, shanmukhi mudra, and unmani mudra.

KAYA MUDRA

These exercises are combined with asanas, breathing techniques, and concentration. Mudras in this category are: vipareeta karani mudra, pashinee mudra, prana mudra, yoga mudra, manduki mudra and tadagi mudra.

BANDHA / LOCK

These exercises combine mudras and bandhas. They charge the system with prana and prepare for the awakening of Kundalini Shakti. Techniques in this category are maha mudra, maha bheda mudra, and maha vedha mudra.

Adhara: these techniques direct the prana from the lower parts of the body to the brain. Techniques that use sexual energy belong to this group and are extremely powerful. Techniques in this category are ashwini mudra and vajroli/sahajoli mudra.

MUDRAS AND OUR ELEMENTS

In the yogic tradition, our hands are like a map of our well-being. Different points in our hands are directly linked to other body parts and our psyche. We stimulate these points and energy paths by making various mudras or hand positions.

Like our surroundings, our physical body comprises five elements: earth, water, fire, air, and ether (space). Many people know the first four elements, but ether (space) is often unknown. Ether (space) is a subtle celestial energy high above our earth. In our body, ether is the space within us at the cellular level.

Imbalances in our elements weaken our immune system, leading to illness in the long run. These deficiencies or inequalities can be corrected by connecting different body parts in a specific way by mudras. Mudras create electromagnetic currents in the body, so-called energy loops.

Each element is also associated with a chakra. When the element is balanced, the chakra is also affected and, in turn, affects the energy (vayu) that belongs to the chakra's area.

Finger	Element / Tattwa	Chakra	Energy / Vayu
Thumb	Fire / agni	Manipura	Samana
Index finger	Air / vayu	Anahata	Prana
Middle finger	Ether / akasha	Vishuddhi	Udana
The ring finger	Earth / prithvi	Mooladhara	Apana
Little finger	Water / apas	Swadhisthana	Vyana

HASTA MUDRA PRANAYAMA
(4 four steps)

SEQUENCE
1. Chin mudra pranayama.

Sit in a comfortable meditation position. Extend the spine and neck. Place your hands, palms facing up, on your knees. Press your thumb against the index finger and let the other fingers point straight out. Sit still, close your eyes, and follow your natural breathing for a few minutes.

Chin mudra opens up the lower lobes of the lungs and stimulates apana vayu (prana that moves down from the navel to the perineum).

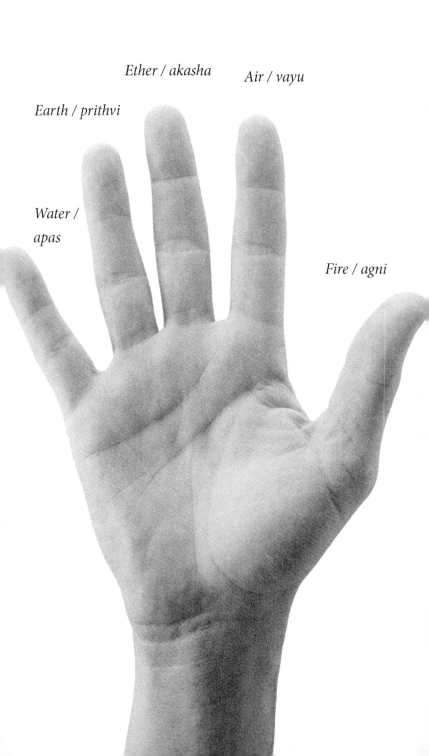

Earth / prithvi

Ether / akasha

Air / vayu

Water / apas

Fire / agni

Physically, it is responsible for the expulsion of toxins in the body.

Sit still and follow the breathing that moves in and out of the nose—two to three minutes.

2. Chin maya mudra pranayama.

Now fold in your fingers without touching your palms. Hold your thumb against your index finger.

Chin maya mudra pranayama opens up the middle lobes of our lungs and stimulates the samana vayu (prana that moves from left to right in the area around the abdomen). Physically, it is responsible for digestion and our ability to assimilate the nutrients in our food. On a subtle level, it affects our ability to absorb (and learn from) life experiences.

Sit still and follow the breathing that moves in and out of the nose—two to three minutes.

3. Aadi mudra pranayama.

Now grab the thumbs with your other fingers and place the fists on the knees with the back of the hand up.

Aadi mudra pranayama opens the upper lobes of our lungs. It stimulates the udana vayu (prana that moves upwards towards the head and outwards in our extremities). Physically, it is responsible for healing and balancing our sense organs. On a subtle level, it is responsible for balancing our perception.

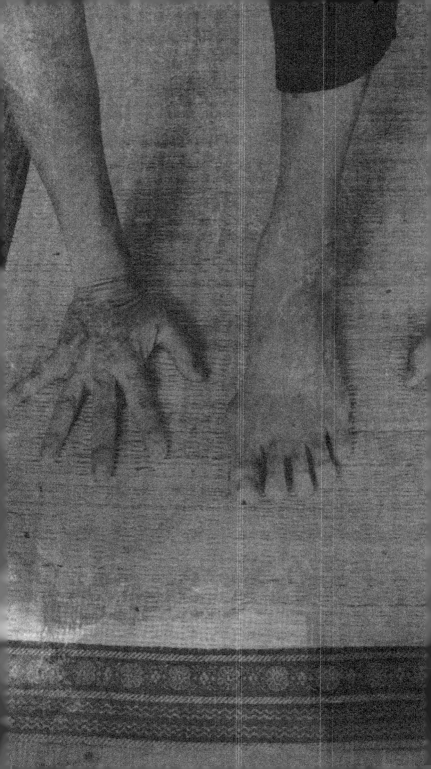

Sit still and follow the breathing that moves in and out of the nose—two to three minutes.

4. Brahma mudra pranayama.

Hold the position of the hands, but turn them so that the wrists are facing upwards and the knuckles are facing each other. Press your hands against your body level with your pelvis.

Brahma mudra pranayama opens up the whole lung. It opens up vyana vayu – the energy that makes us go on a bit longer, the last boost. It balances and starts our other pranas in the body when they become low. It revitalizes the whole system. Sit still and follow the breathing that moves in and out of the nose—two to three minutes.

BANDHA AND GRANTHI

Traditionally, bandhas are classified as part of mudras. In Hatha Yoga Pradipika and old tantric texts, mudras, and bandhas are seen as a whole; they are not separated. Bandhas are linked to mudras and to pranayamas. Bandhas are a technique that creates a unique lock in the body. The word bandha means to hold or lock in Sanskrit. It describes the physical effect created in the body and the retention of prana. Bandhas lock the energy into specific body parts and control the flow to the sushumna nadi to create a spiritual awakening.

Bandhas should be learned as a separate technique before practicing them with mudras and pranayamas.

There are four locking techniques: jalandhara, moola, uddiyana, and maha bandha. Maha is a combination of the first three. These three bandhas directly impact our three mental points (granthis) in the body. Moola bandha is associated with Brahma granthi, uddiyana bandha with Vishnu granthi and jalandhara bandha with Rudra granthi. Granthis prevents the flow of prana and sushumna nadi and inhibits the flow of our chakras and Kundalini Shakti.

Brahma granthi is the first knot linked to Mooladhara and Swadhistana chakra. These are connected to our survival instincts and desires. When you get past the Brahma granthi, Kundalini energy receives an opportunity to wander up and past the Mooladhara and Swadhistana chakra without being drawn back by the instinctive traits of our personality.

The second knot is Vishnu granthi. It is linked to Manipura and Anahata chakra. These two chakras are connected to our emotional and mental sides. Manipura chakra controls our energy body (pranamaya kosha) and affects digestion and metabolism. Anahata controls our mental body (manomaya kosha). Together, the two affect our physical body – annamaya kosha. To transcend Vishnu granthi is no longer bound to physical, mental, and emotional desires. Relationships and energies take on a different character and meaning and are no longer limited to one's wants and needs.

The last knot is Rudra granthi, linked to Vishuddhi and Ajna chakra. Vishuddhi and Ajna control our body of intuition (vijnamaya kosha). When you get past the Rudra granthi, identifying with the ego stops. The experience of unmanifested consciousness appears in the Ajna and Sahasrara chakras.

SHATKARMAS

In the old Upanishads, you can read about Hatha yoga and how it is built up of shatkarmas – purification techniques. Shat means six and karma action. Shatkarmas consists of six different purification techniques. The purpose of Hatha yoga and shatkarmas is to create a balance between ida and pingala nadi, our two most crucial prana in the body, and thus also a balance and purity both physically and mentally.

Shatkarmas are also used to balance the three doshas: vata, pitta, and kapha. According to both Hatha yoga and Ayurveda, an imbalance in the doshas causes illness. The techniques are also used before pranayamas and other more advanced yoga techniques to cleanse the body of toxins and to promote a safe and successful development purely spiritually.

Refrain from attempting to learn the techniques from a book. Seek instructions from a competent teacher who has adequate experience in the field.

Shatkarmas includes the following different techniques:

1. NETI
It is a process where you clean the nasal passages. The techniques are called jala neti and sutra neti.

2. DHAUTI
A series of purification techniques are divided into three main groups: assume dhauti (internal purification), sirshadhauti (purification of the head), and hrid dhauti (purification of the neck). These techniques cleanse the entire nutrient tract from the mouth to the rectum. There are four different techniques:

1.) Shankhaprakshalana and laghooshankhaprakshalana, which cleanse the intestines.

2.) Agnisar kriya, which activates the digestive fire.

3.) Kunjal, where one cleanses the abdomen with the help of water.

4.) Vatsara dhauti, where one cleanses the intestines with air.

3. NAULI
A method to massage and strengthen the abdominal muscles.

4. BASTI
Techniques to clean the colon.

5. KAPALBHATI
Breathing technique to clean the frontal part of the brain.

6. TRATAKA
It's a technique to develop concentration power by focusing on a point or an object. Many tantric yogis believe it is the most powerful method of obtaining siddhis (paranormal abilities).

The six shatkarmas consist of different variations of exercises. Advice and contraindications should be adhered to. Only jala neti (nasal rinsing) and trataka are recommended during pregnancy. While shatkarmas are cleansing and invigorating, they are not the primary purpose of the techniques. Shatkarmas are done to promote the health of those who practice yoga and to awaken and direct the energies in the body and mind safely so they do not flow the wrong way. People suffering from any medical illness should consult a competent teacher before exercising.

JALA NETI / NOSE RINSE

Jala neti is a purification technique all yogis practice before each yoga session. Jala neti cleanses the nasal passages and sinuses from mucus and contaminants. The air can then flow freely through the nose. It counteracts respiratory tract illnesses and promotes healthy ears, eyes, and throat. Tensions in the face are released. It has a calming effect on the brain. Anxiety, anger, and depression are relieved. Jala neti stimulates nerve endings in the nose and promotes the sense of smell. A balance is created between the right and left nostrils and the right and left sides of the brain; it, in turn, creates a balance and harmony between the body and the mind. The most important thing is that jala neti helps awaken Ajna chakra.

"WHO AM I?

AM I MY BODY, OR CAN I EXPERIENCE IT?

AM I MY THOUGHTS, OR DO I HEAR THEM?

AM I MY FEELINGS, OR DO I FEEL THEM?

AM I MY INTUITION, OR DO I SENSE IT?

WHO AM I, I CANNOT BE TWO?

I AM THE BEING, THE CONSCIOUSNESS,
THE ONE WHO EXPERIENCES EVERYTHING.
IN MYSELF BUT ALSO AROUND

I'M THAT, IT'S ME. OM TAT TVASI"

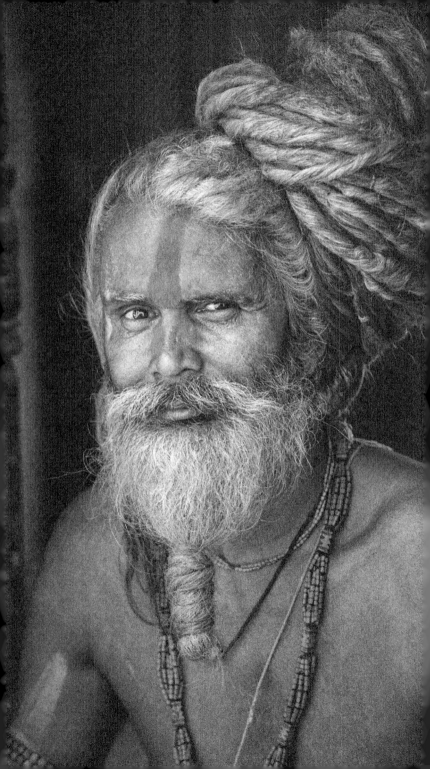

Raja
YOGA

YOGA AS MEDITATION!

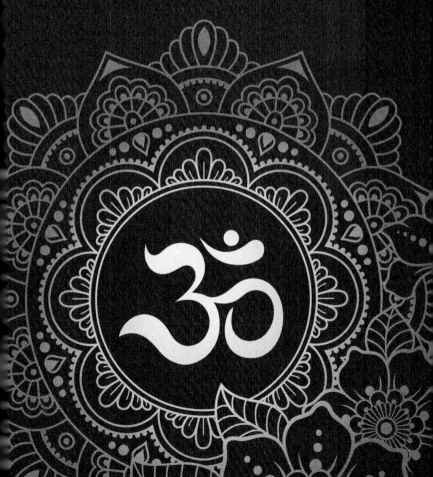

RAJA YOGA

SHIVA AND SHAKTI. YOGA PHILOSOPHY'S TWO PRINCIP-LES – CONSCIOUSNESS AND ENERGY, MAN, AND WOMAN

CLASSICAL YOGA & ITS PHILOSOPHY

In classical yoga and its yoga philosophy, Prakriti (Shakti) is described as cosmic energy. It is the original essence behind everything we can experience, rough and subtle. Prakriti is not in solid form; nothing can be "touched." Prakriti acts as a tool for Purusha (Shiva). Our mind is a result of Prakriti. For consciousness to be able to experience and ex-pand itself, Prakriti is needed. Without Prakriti, consciousness cannot become self-aware.

The qualities of Prakriti are what build up our bodies and our world. It carries karma and coexists through which living beings come into existence and shapes our senses.

Prakriti consists of three qualities – sattva, rajas, and tamas. These three qualities are a basis for the other elements.

PRAKRITI	PURUSHA
All experiences.	*The experience.*
Manifested.	*Unmanifest.*
Background to everything.	*Eternal subject.*
Materially and mentally.	*Infinite amount.*

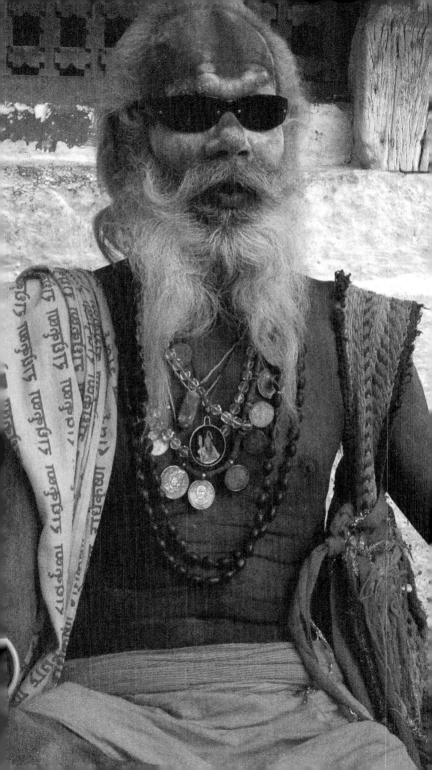

THREE PRINCIPLES BUILD A COSMOS

Thus, our world is built from these three principles – in varying combinations, rajas, tamas, and sattva. The interactions between these gunas govern the cosmos, society, and every human being.

Two primary "laws" describe the interaction between these three works. The first is the "law of alternation," meaning they are in constant motion and collaborate. In sattva, rajas and tamas also exist. In rajas, tamas and sattva live and in tamas, rajas and sattva live. They work together all the time.

The second is the "law of continuity." By this, it means that when a guna has become dominant, it tends to be so for some time.

In yoga, a sattvic state is seen as something of a higher quality, which causes us to develop spiritually. Yoga practice consists of two steps. To create a sattvic condition and then go beyond this condition. This means that we should first purify the body and mind and then go beyond the body and mind and experience our true nature beyond all manifestation. There is also a hidden, mysterious knowledge tradition about activating our chakra system that we will go through later. The fundamental pre-condition for the chakra system to be activated is that the sushumna is open, and that is only when you are in a sattvic state. In scientific terms, these three gunas are described as:

SATTVA
Pure vibration / balance.

RAJAS
Movement.

TAMAS
Inertia / slow / immobility.

One talks about three human characters. The guna that dominates us determines what character we have. You should know the different personality traits and adapt the yoga practice accordingly.

If you are tamasic or slow, it is good with a dynamic form of yoga where you get the activity going in the body and, in this way, can create balance. Hatha yoga or physical work suits tamasic people.

If you are rajasic or mobile, you often need help with concentrating. Here, it is essential to have a lot of relaxation but to relax and release tension, a dynamic form of yoga is also required. You exhaust your body and mind to be able to relax more easily. Hatha yoga, Bhakti yoga (e.g., kirtan), Japa yoga, and Karma yoga suit rajasic people.

If you are sattvic or balanced, it is easy to focus and concentrate and well suited to Satsang and studies. But even if you are sattvic, you must work with the body. It's to create balance in the already balanced thought activity.

A rule to follow is that inertia is balanced with movement, and movement is balanced with even more movement. We always start with the outer, the surface, our body, and go inward, deeper, balancing and activating. We always start with the movement. Always.

ISHVARA
Yoga is a practical method based on the Samkhya philosophy, but unlike Samkhya, yoga's view of creation is theistic.

In classical yoga, the God or creator is called Ishvara in Sanskrit. Ishvara is said to be the force that creates, maintains, and destroys the world through the three forms: Brahma, Vishnu, and Shiva, as well as their female counterparts Saraswati, Lakshmi, and Kali.

Although Ishvara is very similar to our Western God, they differ in that Ishvara works through different gods and goddesses; it has different shapes and manifestations. Ishavara can also be worshiped in a female form and is then called Ishvari. It's common in many yoga traditions, especially those of tantric origin. Ishvari is then equated with Shakti.

Ishvara is not described separately in Samkhya, but in many yoga traditions, Ishvara is described as Purusha (Shiva in tantrism).

DARSHANS

Vedas are writings composed of rishis (sight / medium) and yogis about 5000 years ago (they can also be much older). These describe the wisdom behind the cosmic mind, which is said to be the origin of the universe and creation. From the beginning, these writings have been passed on orally and then written down. Yoga has its roots in Vedic teachings. Rishis gave Vedic knowledge a practical form, yoga.

From the Vedas, six philosophical paths / views were developed, shad darshans, which means "six ways of seeing" or "six ways of insight." Ass described by Patanjali in the Yoga Sutras, classical yoga is one of these.

Hiranyagarbha, the sun god, and the cosmic creator, is traditionally said to be the creator of the yoga system.

The six Vedic / spiritual paths:

1. *Nyaya – logical doctrine – Gautama.*

2. *Vaisheshika – atomic doctrine – Kannada.*

3. *Samkhya – the doctrine of the cosmic principle – Kapila.*

4. *Yoga – the doctrine of yoga – Hiranyagarbha.*

5. *Purva Mimamsa / Vedanta – ritual doctrine – Jasmine.*

6. *Yttara Mimamsa / Vedanta – theological doctrine – Badarayana.*

Nyaya and Vaisheshka's teachings are based on logical philosophy. These can be compared to Plato's philosophy as we know it in the West.

Samkhya is the philosophy behind yoga and Ayurveda. It is based on a scientific approach that explores our inner and outer reality. Samkhya describes tattwas / cosmic principles that one tries to gain insight into and experience with the help of various yogic exercises. Samkhya describes the knowledge behind the different elements, and yoga is a technique that should purify and balance the corresponding components in ourselves.

Purva Mimamsa refers to Karma yoga, which acts as a channel for the creative energy of the universe. You work and contribute with selfless services / work to people and society. It is also part of focusing on a prayer or a mantra during the work. It cleanses both the mind and the body and is a good preparation for meditation.

Uttara Mimamsa is the system where you go in-depth for the Vedic texts. One discusses God, the soul, the absolute, and their interaction.

AUM

A common symbol in yoga is Om. The emblem is made up of three syllables that together form a whole. Sanskrit's vowel "o" consists of "a + u." So, Om can also be spelled as Aum. It represents the trinity of our existence.

The symbol A-u-m consists of three "curves," a semicircle and a point. The most significant "curve" at the bottom refers to our waking state when our consciousness is turned outwards and when we take in the environment with the help of our sense organs. It's called jagarat. It is symbolized by the most significant "curve" because it is our most common state. Beta waves dominate in this state – we are aware.

The second largest curve at the top of the symbol refers to deep sleep and our unconscious state. We neither dream nor feel desire. This condition is called sushputi. Delta waves dominate in this state – we are unconscious.

The slightest curve between these two refers to our dream state, swapana. Here, the consciousness is turned inwards; you experience the world with closed eyes. Theta waves dominate in this state—the experience of the subconscious.

The point in the symbol refers to our fourth state of consciousness which in Sanskrit is called turiya. Here, we look neither outwards nor inwards but are in pure being. That is the unmanifest state of Purusha. Alpha waves dominate in this state – we are superconscious.

The semicircle refers to the Maya, which separates the point turiya from the "three curves." Maya symbolizes what hinders our ability to experience our true nature. That the semicircle is just half tells us that Maya cannot change the experience that exists within us, the stillness / being / bliss. Maya can only decide what is manifested.

Aum thus symbolizes the manifested and the unmanifested. What we can see and cannot see represents the trinity of our existence. The

Aum

sound and vibrations that occur when we sound Om / Aum affect our whole being on all these levels and are a powerful mantra. It permeates our entire interior and makes us vibrate in step with the universe. Aum – the sound / vibration of the cosmos and creation.

VIVEKA

Patanjali (the author of the Yoga Sutras) describes Viveka, i.e., discernment. The purpose of eight-step yoga (classical yoga) is precisely to develop Viveka within us, i.e., awareness, which is a prerequisite for understanding the goal of yoga.

It requires a sharp ability to pay attention and distinguish the experiencer from the experience, see what our true identity is and what is perishable. We also need intense attention to know the reason for our ignorance of this – i.e., to miss what is changeable for immutable, to forget what is destructive for improvement, to ignore desires for need, to identify with the ego instead of the true self.

VAIRAGYA

When we developed Viveka, a change took place in us. We begin to let go of our desires. It is called Vairagya. We no longer cling to what will disappear anyway. When we understand the principle of transience, we can take a more understanding approach to life's worries and troubles. If you read about the yoga philosophy, you know that Buddha was enlightened in India at about the same time as Patanjali, where he took his inspiration for the eightfold path. People often talk about Buddhism as a cousin of the yoga philosophy. Many of the ideas are similar.

RAGA

Everything we experience and "take in" from our surroundings happens with our senses. Through our eyes (sight), ears (hearing), nose (scent), tongue (taste), body / skin (feeling), and mind (thoughts, feelings, images). They can then be divided into comfortable, uncomfortable, and neutral experiences. Most often, we want to re-experience the comfortable experiences and provide enjoyment. We want to recreate these experiences time and time again. It is called raga.

Events that we experience as painful and unpleasant, we want to avoid. Most of the time, we try to find what gives us pleasure and avoid what is painful. It creates dissatisfaction and a divided mind. We need more than what is. We do not accept life for what it is.

DRASHTA BHAVA

In yoga, we create a third approach called drashta bhava. It can be translated as "witness attitude." Here, we have a neutral and relaxed attitude to our negative and positive thoughts. This approach, with Viveka, leads to liberation, the ultimate purpose of yoga. To be free from desire, not to be controlled by ideas and feelings. To be happy with what is – whatever it looks like right now. To accept what we cannot change.

CURRENT CLASSICAL YOGA:

SATYANANDA YOGA

Today, classical yoga is taught through, among other things, Satyananda yoga. It is a system developed by Swami Satyananda Saraswati. They use ancient and traditional techniques: Asanas to balance body and mind, pranayamas to work with the energy body, and meditation to calm and focus the mind. Tradition teaches the general yogic lifestyle to the "ordinary modern man" and the more devoted practitioner. Eve-

ryone can take part in yoga. Jnana, Bhakti, and Karma yoga, among others, are also part of the Satyananda system.

In Satyananda yoga, one considers the whole being of man, not just the body. You want to give the individual an opportunity to discover and develop all aspects of one's personality with the help of yoga. It is believed that change happens with regular practice, under entire presence and awareness, not by pushing the body or mind beyond its means.

SRI SWAMI SIVANANDA SARASWATI

Swami Satyananda's guru and perhaps India's most famous yoga personality – Sri Swami Sivananda Saraswati, was born in Pattamadai in 1887. Sivananda worked as a doctor before quitting to find his guru in the Himalayas. He settled in Rishikesh, where he was initiated into dashnami sannyasa by his guru Swami Vishwananda Saraswati in 1924. Over the years, he and his disciples wrote hundreds of books and articles on yoga and spirituality to spread the knowledge to the general public. Sri Swami Sivananda wanted to give the needy the knowledge that could help them, whether it was about improving physical health, creating peace of mind, or developing spiritually. It still characterizes Satyananda yoga today.

SWAMI SATYANANDA SARASWATI

Swami Satyananda Saraswati was born in Almora in 1923. At nineteen, he met Sukhman Giri, from Juna-Akhara, a Tantric yogini from Nepal. From her, he learned, among other things, the Tantric nyasa techniques, which he developed further with Swami Sivananda. Nyasa is a technique for raising awareness by placing different energies in the body parts. From there, he created the world-famous deep relaxation yoga nidra. In 1943, he met his guru, Swami Sivananda, and was initiated into dashnami sannyasa in 1947. After serving his guru's mission for twelve years, Satyanada began his journey through India as an ascetic to discover the needs of society. In 1956, Swami Satyananda founded the International Yoga Fellowship and, in 1963, the Bihar School Of Yoga, hoping to spread ancient yogic knowledge to all corners of the world. For twenty years, Swami Satyananda traveled worldwide, spreading the wisdom of yoga. He and his disciples also authored over eighty yoga, Tantra, and spirituality books. In 1984 he founded the "Yoga Research Foundation" and "Sivananda Math" to help disadvantaged people.

YOGA FORMS

In Satyananda yoga, the following forms of yoga are applied:

JNANA YOGA

The path of spiritual insight is where one, through intellectual and theoretical knowledge, studies life and tries to distinguish the truth from the perishable. This path is suitable for theoretically inclined people.

BHAKTI YOGA

The path of devotion and love consists of song, dance, or meditation on an image of a guru or the divine. The practicer strives to create a personal relationship with the sacred and merge with it.

KARMA YOGA

Selfless service is where you help others and society without taking advantage of it or shining in the glory.

HATHA YOGA

Here, you want to balance and strengthen the physical and mental body as a preparation for the more advanced exercises in Kundalini yoga. Asanas, pranayamas, bandhas and shatkarmas are used.

RAJA YOGA – CLASSIC YOGA

The path of meditation. It refers to the system described in Patanjali's Yoga Sutras.

KRIYA YOGA

Satyananda taught Kriya yoga based on the secret exercises of yoga and tantra shastras. Kriya means "activity" or "movement" and refers to the natural movement of consciousness. Kriya yoga does not stop the movements of the mind but instead creates an action in the mind that leads to a conscious increase and awakening. There are seventy kriyas, of which twenty are best known and used.

THE TRADITIONS

In addition to the yogic tradition, Satyananda yoga also includes the Tantric and Vedic traditions.

Tantra refers to practical exercises that expand the human consciousness and the awakening of Kundalini Shakti. The principle behind the tantric system is that one uses the material world and its experiences to become enlightened.

Tantra is often described as a sexual tradition where you want to enhance the sexual experience. Originally, Tantra was intended to awaken Kundalini Shakti, a dormant potential force in man.

"I'M WAITING TO LEAVE THIS BODY, BUT I'M NOT GOING TO LEAVE IT UNTIL I GET MY RETURN TICKET. I DO NOT WANT EMANCIPATION, MOKSHA, OR ANY PERSONAL SATISFACTION WHICH COMES WITH SPIRITUAL ENLIGHTENMENT. MY AIM AND ASPIRATION IN THIS AND IN ALL FUTURE LIVES IS TO HELP OTHERS. TO WIPE THE TEARS OF SUFFERING AND PAIN FROM THE EYES OF EVERY PERSON WHO IS SEEKING SOLACE, PEACE, PLENTY AND PROSPERITY. THAT IS THE ONLY PURPOSE OF MY LIFE"

(SWAMI SATYANANDA SARASWATI)

There are many tantric paths, and the common denominator of these paths is the use of mantras, yantras (concentration symbols used to liberate consciousness), chakras, mandalas (discovering macrocosm in microcosm), tapasya (self-purification), Raja yoga, pranayama, shakti-pat (power transmission) and Tantric initiations to reach awakening. Tantrism advocates a life in which the qualities of the intellect and the heart are exploited. To discern and focus with the help of the mind and to see and experience with the spirit the unseen, the cosmic conscious-ness beyond the material.

The Vedic tradition is one of the oldest preserved spiritual traditions in existence. It advocates the divine as the ultimate truth and life accor-dingly in the material world.

Central to Vedic doctrine is that God is constantly present, omniscient, and omnipotent, while the individual is only an actor. To experience the reality that is Satyam (truth), Shivam (favorable), and Sundaram (beautiful), the individual should live a life where one strives to harmo-nize thoughts, behavior, and actions: a meditative contemplation, belief in God and oneself. Living in harmony with, and being grateful for, the environment and nature and experiencing unity are the foundations of the Vedic tradition.

All the Vedic and Tantric traditions are held together by yoga. Yoga is the practical principle of the spiritual paths that lead to increased awareness and self-insight.

RAJA YOGA – THE ROYAL PATH

Patanjali never gave his system any specific title. He called it yoga. In time, however, his method became known as Patanjali's and classical yoga. Patanjali's yoga is one of the different forms of Raja yoga (Raja means royal):

Kundalini yoga (also called Laya yoga).
Kriya yoga.
Yoga mantra.
Dhyana yoga.
Patanjali yoga.

Raja yoga is the doctrine of the mind. You explore your inner world to exploit your strength and knowledge here. Raja yoga teaches different methods to create a focused mind. It is based on mental discipline.

Patanjali defined his method as "elimination of mental fluctuations" – Yoga chitta vritti nirodha. Usually translated to – when the mind is still, yoga occurs. The mind can be described as the visible part of the pure consciousness and divided into the conscious, the subconscious, and the unconscious. Patanjali's definition means yoga is the control of the pattern of consciousness.

VIYOGA
Who is experiencing this?

Most people know that yoga means union, but in the Yoga Sutras, Patanjali describes yoga as a separation process. It can be explained by the Samkhya philosophy, which is the foundation of the Yoga Sutras.

Samkhya divides existence and individuality into two aspects we have touched on – Purusha and Prakriti. The existence and the individual are created when these two merge. Purusha refers to the one who sees / experiences drashta. Prakriti refers to the seen, drishya.

91

Practicing yoga and its process leads to yoga, a separation between the one who experiences and the seen. It leads to yoga, the association that is the very development of yoga, the culmination. At first, Purusha and Prakriti must be separated from each other, and then it is understood that these are the same.

It can also be described that the pure consciousness (Purusha) is broken down by incorrect identification with mind and body (Prakriti). The purpose of yoga is to release pure consciousness from the mind and body.

The experience of the difference and separation between Purusha and Prakriti leads to the realization that everything is the same.

EIGHT STEPS / ASHTANGA

Patanjali describes a series of techniques that have a slow and harmonizing effect on our minds and perceptions. The most crucial thing in Patanjali's system is described in the eight steps. The first five steps are preparatory to the other three steps and belong to bhairanga / outer yoga. Ashtanga means eight different steps and should not be confused in this context with the modern Ashtanga yoga developed by yoga master Shri K. Pattabhi Jois.

You must not see the first five steps as a staircase; you can also see it as a wheel where you influence others by working with one step.

1. Yama – is about moral discipline in social life.

2. Niyama – is about restraint on a personal level.

3. Asana – sitting position/body position. It refers to the correct meditation position / lotus position so that you can remain immobile during the meditation and are not distracted by the physical body.

4. Pranayama – respiratory regulation / control of prana / kumbhaka. By controlling breathing, you can control the life force/prana in the body and calm the mind.

5. Pratyahara – removal of sensory impressions. By blocking sensory impressions, one is not distracted by the external environment.

The last three steps belong to antharanga / inner yoga. One must have absorbed the first five preparatory steps to develop in-depth and succeed with these steps. The steps before pratyahara gradually dissolve external obstacles in life, while the exercises after eliminating thoughts and inner images so that the mind is still. Ida (our inner world) becomes balanced with pingala (our outer world) so that the sushumna (our supersensible world) begins to exist during samadhi.

6. Dharana – concentration. Focus on a meditation object.

7. Dhyana – meditation. After a more extended concentration, you naturally sink into meditation. Here, one is fulfilled by the meditation object.

8. Samadhi – liberation / ecstasy / superconscious. Meditation eventually leads to samadhi. Here, the movements of the mind have stopped, and you become one with the meditation object and experience powerful ecstasy / joy. There are twelve stages of samadhi; the last stage leads to the liberation of the cycle of rebirth.

The eight steps gradually balance our five koshas (shells): Annamaya,
pranamaya, manomaya, vijnamaya and anandamaya. The boundary
between the shells is loosened from the coarsest – the body, annamaya
kosha, to the most subtle, our innermost interior – anandamaya kosha.

YAMA
Satya – truth, to be true to oneself and others.
Ahimsa – do not be involved in the killing.
Asteya – do not steal, do not take more than you need, and share.
Aparighara – not to be greedy, to live materially.
Brahmacharya – chastity. To live ascetically, not indulge in pleasures as
they are considered to distract one from reaching the goal of yoga.

NIYAMA
Saucha – purity of speech and action, sensory impressions (media,
television, radio), food, hygiene.
Santosha – contentment, to be happy with what you have. If we focus
on what we do not have, we create even more emptiness within our-
selves. If we focus on shortages, we get even more shortages (the law of
attraction).
Tapas – self-discipline, hardening of the inner fire.
Swadhyaya – studies.
Ishwara pranidhara – means to surrender one's will to the higher will.

Yamas thus create a balance in our interaction with the outside world,
and niyamas harmonize our inner feelings. These rules are designed
to balance our external actions with our internal settings. The mind
affects our external actions at the same time as our external actions
affect the mind. If our actions are not good, the mind will also be
negatively affected, which creates a vicious circle as a distracted mind

creates less good actions. Yamas and niyamas are designed to break the vicious circle. It can be challenging to follow these rules, but even a small change does a lot to balance the mind.

PATANJALIS YOGA SUTRAS

Patanjali's work consists of one hundred and ninety-six sutras. The word sutra itself is often incorrectly translated as verse. The actual translation is "to thread in a row," which also describes how the sutras are linked to each other and carry an underlying continuity. The work is considered the most accurate and scientific yogic text ever written.

Who Patanjali was and when he lived is still being determined. It has also yet to be possible to decide when his work was written and whether he was a man or a woman. There is still some evidence that he must have lived about 300-400 years BC.

Patanjali gives us a range of techniques that gradually balance and harmonize our minds. The unique thing is that Patanjali does not describe a single yoga position as we are usually used to. Here, instead, the focus is on yoga from a moral perspective. When Patanjali talked about asana, he referred to a steady and comfortable position to sit and meditate in.

Many great masters and yogis have translated and interpreted Patanjali's work.

The following sutras are some of the most important to know:

3:2
Cause of suffering.
Avidyāsmitārāgadveṣābhiniveśāh kleśāh
Avidy: erroneous knowledge, asmit: I-experience, raga: liking, dves: reluctance, abhiniveh: fear of death, klesah: suffering.

Klesha is the suffering that is present in everyone. According to Patanjali, the basis of all suffering is incorrect identification with the experience. Everyone carries a subconscious suffering, but we are seldom aware of it in our daily lives; all the musts and chores block the experience of it.

We rarely become aware of our fear of dying, even if it is in our sub- conscious. The fear of dying is the basis of our most incredible suffering. Kleshas is like a chain of misfortune that begins with our ignorance of our true nature based on our ego. We try to find pleasure and avoid suffering, creating fear and tension. The solution to being free from suffering is meditation.

4:2

The root cause.

Avidyākṣetramuttareṣām prasuptatanuvichchhinnodārāṇām

Avidya: incorrect knowledge, ksetram: area, uttaresam: of the fol- lowing, prasupta: dormant, tanu: weak, vichchhinna: alternating, udaranam: fully active.

Avidya is the field of dormant, weak, alternating, and fully active states of kleshas.

Avidya is the basis of the other four kleshas: asmita, raga, dweshta, and abhinivesha. These are either dormant, weak, alternating, or fully active. When we learn to deal with avidya, we can also learn to deal with the other four kleshas more easily. Avidya is about the ignorance of our true nature. We must learn to control the kleshas to return to our true nature.

5:2

Incorrect knowledge.

Anityāśuchiduhkhānātmasu nityaśuchisukhātmakhyātiravidyā

Anitya: not eternal, asuchi: unclean, duhkha: pain, natmasu: not atman, nitya: eternal, suchi: pure, sukha: goodness, atma: self, khyati: knowledge, avidya: erroneous knowledge.

Avidya means that one confuses the eternal, impure, and evil with the infinite, pure, good, and atman.

Avidaya is about ignorance of our true nature and identification with the body. We are free from Avidaya by developing our discernment, viveka. Through viveka, we can distinguish between our body and atman, our inner true self.

Avidaya is also called Maya. In a cosmic context, it is called maya, and on an individual level, it is called avidaya.

6:2

Separation, I, ego.

Dṛgdarśanaśaktyorekātmatevāsmitā

Drg: Purusha, the power of consciousness, darsana: the seen, saktyoh: of the two forces, ekatmate: identity, eva: like that, dodge: I-feeling.

Asmita can be described as an identification of Purusha as a Buddhi.

Asmita means that our inner consciousness, our true self, is mixed with our existence, body, actions, and mind. When our true self is expressed through the body, actions, and mind, it is called asmita. Purusha is identified by its means of expression / instrument. It can be expressed in different ways, as identification with the body or in a more intellectually developed person as identification with the more developed sensory functions. Our ability to see, think, and hear comes from Purusha, expressed through our senses. When we mix these, it is called Asmita.

Shakti, the power of Purusha, lies behind the ability to think, see, etc., mixed with the actual means / instruments with which these are expressed. By meditating, we can realize that Purusha is not a part of the body or the intellect (Buddhi). We come across Asmita.

7:2

Attraction, I want.

Sukhānuśayå rāgah

Sukha: satisfaction, anusayl: accompanying, ragah: pleasure, liking.

Raga is the pleasure created by satisfaction.

Raga is about the mind constantly wanting to recreate a previous experience of pleasure.

8:2

Repulsion, I do not want.

Duhkahānuśayå dveṣah

Duhka: pain, anusayl: accompanying, dvesah: reluctance.

Dwesha is our reluctance to experience pain.

Dwesha is the opposite of raga. You want to avoid what creates discomfort. Raga and dwesha keep us in the lower stages of consciousness. As long as raga and dwesha rule over us, we do not develop spiritually.

To like something also means you do not want the opposite of what you like. So raga and dwesha are not opposites but two sides of the mind. Dwesha is what affects us most negatively because it is based on a lot of hatred. The elimination of dweshta allows for more profound meditation and the natural elimination of raga.

9:2

Fear of dying.

Svarasavāhī viduṣo ´pi tathārūdho ´bhiniveśah

Svarasavahi: persistence of self, vidusah: of the learned, api: also, tatha: like it, rudhah: dominant, abhinivesah: fear of death.

Abnivecha is the hope of being able to live and be maintained by one's power, even among scholars.

It is the most dominant klesha. All individuals experience fear of dying. It is an innate, inherent force that exists naturally in us, a self-preservation drive. As children, we do not share this the same way, but the older we get, the more aware we become of it.

In those who have developed viveka, abhinivecha is almost eliminated. Still, in most people, it can be seen in its most active form, which can also lead to fear and panic in, for example, a severe illness. In ancient Indian texts, one can read about the cause of abhnivecha, which is identifying with the body.

11:2

Meditation – the solution to the elimination of kleshas.

Dhyānaheyāstadvṛttayah

Dhyana: meditation, heyah: reduces, tadvrttayah: modification, change.

The modification of the kleshas can be reduced through meditation.

We can learn to understand our fears / kleshas by observing the mind. These exist in our subconscious as well as in our conscious mind to varying degrees. In our normal daily state, we rarely see the character of the kleshas. We can not eliminate the kleshas with the help of the intellect; it can only be done with meditation.

It takes a sharp ability to pay attention to become aware of how kleshas look in ourselves. For example, we may believe that we are not afraid of death even though we unconsciously are. We do not see it. Even individuals who have been engaged in spiritual development for a long time – who for several years have experienced peace and thought they are free from samskaras and kleshas, can suddenly experience obstacles and failure. The kleshas' seed, root, and cause remain and come up to the surface. You need to practice the whole yoga system in-depth to eliminate kleshas. Yamas, niyamas and Kriya yoga. By dhyana, i.e., to observe what happens to us mentally. It is done by paying attention to our good and bad thoughts and letting them surface. In the long run, it prevents kleshas from manifesting in the most active form, which creates suffering and fear in our daily lives. In this case, one does not refer to "object focus" when discussing dhyana but assumes mouna, i.e., one focuses on how kleshas look and its character and strength.

By focusing and observing, vrittis is weakened. It explains why medita-tion has such a calming effect on us. During meditation, our uncons-cious fears can surface so that we become aware of them. Tensions caused by our fears / kleshas are weakened, and we can relax. A feeling of inner harmony arises.

When our fears / kleshas have taken on a more latent form, we should, through our discernment / viveka, try to find the cause of the fear. You may be dependent on something, or you want to be successful.

Dhyana (Raja yoga) and Viveka (Jnana yoga) are thus two essential tools in eliminating our fears / kleshas. To prevent being drawn back to the unconscious state again – when one experiences risk becoming too challenging to deal with – Karma and Bhakti yoga can be beneficial.

2:1

What is yoga?

Yogaschitta vṛitti nirodhah

Yogah: yoga, chitta: consciousness, vritti: patterns, movements, nirodhah: blocked – still.

When the movements of the mind are still, yoga occurs.

Chitta refers to the mind, the individual consciousness on the conscious, unconscious, and subconscious planes.

Nirodhah aims to block the movements of the mind, the pattern of consciousness, not the mind or consciousness itself. It happens automatically when we sleep. The normal flow of vrittis is stopped, and we are moved to another state of consciousness. We experience other things, people, events, and places. With this, we can understand that within us, something exists independently of our body, mind, and life energy/prana, something utterly different from any of these. This "something" is consciousness, a constant and uninterrupted state.

Vritti can be translated as "circular," which describes chitta's movements. They are like rings on the water.

So, what is yoga? Yoga is to calm the movements of the mind on all planes of consciousness. It is not about shutting down or shielding oneself from the external impressions we encounter daily. We want to get past the experiences and visions that our consciousness creates during deep meditation and higher stages of samadhi. When this happens, yoga occurs. It is a prerequisite for the development of human consciousness.

When one ceases to identify with Prakriti, the three gunas develop our consciousness.

They talk about the five different characters of the mind. If you compare these with the Kundalini awakening, you can see that moodha / the sluggish mind is associated with the Mooladhara chakra, where the individual consciousness is dormant.

After practicing specific exercises, the consciousness is stimulated to direct itself to the area around the navel, the Manipura chakra. This state of consciousness is called kshipta and belongs to rajas. Most often, however, it sinks to Mooladhara chakra again and then rises to Swadhisthana chakra, Manipura chakra, and again to Mooladhara chakra. Once consciousness has stabilized in the Manipura chakra for some time – vikshipta, it will steer further through the Anahata chakra and the Vishuddhi chakra to the Ajna chakra. In this state of consciousness – echagrata, the consciousness is focused and concentrated, sattvic. Further, in the Sahasrara chakra, one achieves the state of nirodha beyond the three gunas and sattva.

The interaction between the three gunas governs all functions in our body, mind, and environment. Even though one guna dominates, the other two are always present and affect our consciousness. We should learn to see which guna dominates and how the other two come into play and then learn to balance these to control consciousness.

3:1

When yoga culminates – then the sight is established.

Tadā draṣṭuh svarūpe´vasthānam

Tada: then, drasuh: seeing – answer, upe: the essential nature of one-self, vasthanam: establish, develop.

The seeing develops in its true nature.

Self-awareness, kaivalya, is the very goal of yoga in this context. It develops when the activity of chitta vritti ceases, when the mind is no longer affected by the interaction of the three gunas, and when one stops to identify with the material world.

The insight into our true nature comes from within. It is impossible to create or experience this insight in the state of consciousness where one still identifies with the self, the ego. Reaching this insight takes purity of mind, complete mind control, and freedom from desire.

4:1

What else happens to Purusha?

Vátti sārūpyamitaratra

Vrtti: modification, pattern, syrupy: identification, iterate: another state.

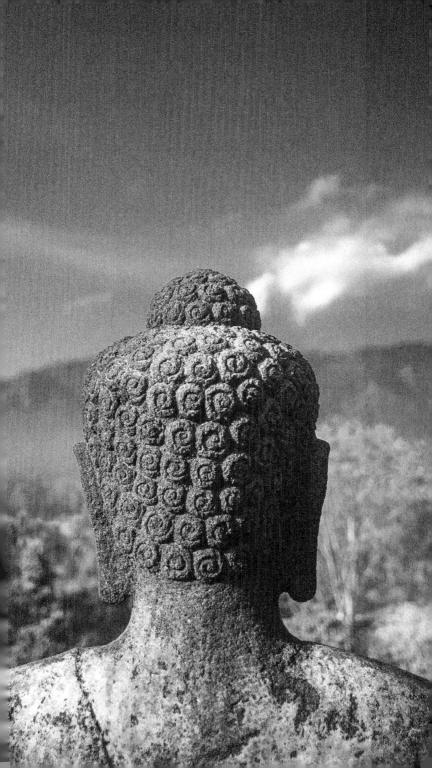

Otherwise, there is an identification with the movements of the mind.

When the movements of the mind, chitta vrittis, are not in the state of nirodha and have not calmed down, Purusha can not become aware of himself. Instead, there is an identification with chitta and its fluctuations.

When there is no awareness of the pure consciousness, Purusha, we identify with the movements of the chitta and are controlled by emotions such as feeling angry, sad, or scared.

Patanjali describes different techniques that are adapted to the different needs of individuals, depending on temperament, to lead chitta to the state of nirodha. It is a prerequisite for Purusha to become aware of its true nature.

5:1
Vrittis – main divisions.
Vṛttayah pañchatayyah kliṣṭāakliṣṭāh
Vrttayah: modification of the mind, pañchatayyah: fivefold, klista: painful, difficult, aklistah: not painful.

The modification of the mind is fivefold; these are either painful or not.

There are five types of vrittis, either painful or non-painful. In total, there are ten types of vrittis. When you experience something pleasant, e.g., looking at a beautiful flower, it is called aklishta. When you experience something painful and uncomfortable, it is called klishta.

According to Patanjali, everything we see, hear, think, and feel is a

106

different formation of the mind. According to the yogic system, all our
thoughts, knowledge, and various planes of consciousness are vital, as
well as our dreams.

6:1

Five types of vrittis.

Pramāṇa-viparyaya-vikalpa-nidrā smṛtayah

Pramana: right knowledge, viparyaya: wrong knowledge, vikalpa:
imagination, nidra: sleep, smrtayah: memory.

The five different patterns of the mind are proper knowledge, wrong
knowledge, imagination, sleep, and memory.

Our mind comprises five types of vrittis: correct knowledge, false know-
ledge, imagination, deep sleep, and memory. These five build up the
mind and shape the three dimensions of the individual consciousness.
All states of mind belong to these five sensory patterns or vrittis (wake-
fulness, dreams, seeing, speaking, hearing, touching, crying, feeling, and
doing).

The ultimate goal of yoga is to break down these manifestations of the
pattern of consciousness, i.e., vrittis.

12:1

The importance of abhyasa and vairagya.

Abhyāsavairāgyābhyām tannirodhah

Abhyasa: continuous practice, vairagyabhyam: through, vairagya, tat:
it, nirodhah: stills.

Calming the five movement patterns of the mind takes place through
regular exercise and vairagya.

Patanjali describes two ways to stop the flow of chitta vrittis. Abhyasa and vairagya. Abhyasa means regular exercise. Vairagya aims at liberation from raga and dweshta, i.e., attraction and reluctance to like / dislike. If you have control over these, meditation will be more accessible.

15:1

A lower state of vairagya.

Dṛṣṭānuśravika-viṣayāvitṛṣṇasya vaśīkāra-sañjñā vairāgyam

Drsta: the seen, anusravika: the heard, visaya: object, vitrsnasya: of the one free from desire, vasikara: control, sañjña: consciousness, vairagyam: absence of desire.

The state of consciousness is when the individual becomes free from the desire to satisfy the mind with what has previously been experienced, and what one has heard of is vairagya.

It is called vairagya when one is free from desire and no longer longs for the pleasures one has experienced. One is free from hunger in the face of all objects of the mind.

It is possible to achieve vairagya even if one lives in a normal society with a family and job. It is not necessary to give up these. However, what you absolutely must give up completely is raga and dweshta.

Vairagya starts from within ourselves, not from outside. It does not matter what clothes you wear or which people you live with. What matters is what kind of attitude you have towards the events and people you meet in life. Vairagya is divided into three stages. In the first step, you are fully aware of the desires and unwillingness that you *carry, and you work to get over raga and dweshsta. In the second stage, some objects of raga and dwehsta have been taken over, but something remains. In the third stage, the mind is entirely free from these, but they can remain latent in the subconscious.*

16:1

A higher state of vairagya.

Tatparam puruṣakhyātergunạvaitṛṣṇyam

Tat: it, param: supreme, purusakhyateh: proper knowledge of Purusha, gunavaitrsnyam: free from the lusts of gunas.

The highest is when one becomes free from the lusts of gunas with the knowledge of Purusha.

Once one has reached this higher state of vairagya, there is no longer a need to experience pleasure and enjoyment, acquire knowledge, or be dependent on sleep. This state of vairagya is achieved when one becomes aware of Purusha.

21:1

The strength of curiosity is faster.

Tảvrasamveḡānāmāsannah

Tlvra: intensity, samvega: curiosity, asannah: close.

Those with intense curiosity and desire, samvega, achieve asamprajnata samadhi soon.

One realizes that everything is perishable, which is a prerequisite for wanting to seek the truth.

23:1

The degree of curiosity and devotion to Ishwara (God).

Mṛdumadhyādhimātratvāt tato'pi viśeṣah

Mrdu: small, madhya: medium, adhimatra: strong, tvat: dependent on, tatopi: even, more than, viseah: specific.

As the desire grows in intensity from being minor to becoming strong, asamprajnata samadhi can be achieved faster. God refers to a superior spiritual consciousness. It is neither physical nor mental but only spiritual—the highest manifested consciousness in man. According to Patanjali, if you find it challenging to develop spiritually through the techniques described, you can also do so by devoting yourself intensely to God.

28:1

Sadhana for Ishvara.

Tajjapastadarthabhāvanam

Tat: it, japa: repetition of the word, tat: it, artha: meaning, bhavanam: filled with mental.

To recite Aum and fill the mind with its meaning.

What separates Ishwara from man is that man is the manifested state of consciousness, while Ishwara is the highest state. The displayed condition continues to be manifested through rebirths and incarnations and takes shape in various bodies, such as humans and animals. It forms a finer and more developed body when it reaches the highest stage of evolution. Ishvara is beyond the manifestation of life and death and is, therefore, seen as the guru of the departed masters and prophets.

One must be able to reach Ishwara by thinking or speaking and by our intellect. Feeling and experiencing are two different things. The Indian philosophical system is divided into tattwa chintana, a reflection of the highest consciousness, and tattwa darshan, an experience of the highest consciousness. India's six intelligent systems are based on tattwa chintana, i.e., knowledge. Tattwa darshan's experience develops through yoga, Bhakti, mystery, and occult rituals.

Aum is like a means of expression for Ishwara, which is otherwise wholly formless. It is described in yantra, mantra, and Tantra. These three are expressions of the supernatural. Mantra is like a term in the form of sound. Pure consciousness is denoted and described in terms of the power of sound. In Tantra, there is symbolism in the form of humans and animals. Yantra is a mental symbol. Aum is both a mantra and a yantra. It is not Tantra, as it must have a human form and have no sound.

We cannot experience Ishwara with our eyes or ears, but we experience it within ourselves using a mantra. Aum denotes Ishvara.

The meditation becomes complete by constantly repeating the words Aum and dhyana about their meaning. Japa is not enough but must go hand in hand with meditation. Patanjali recommends that during the rehearsal of Aum, one should be aware of japa and its significance. Therefore, it is essential to understand the meaning of Aum. It is made up of three letters A-u-m. A relates to the world we perceive with our senses and body. U relates to the subconscious mind. M relates to the unconscious mind. By understanding this and repeating the mantra, one can change the three states of manifested consciousness, go beyond these, and finally reach the fourth and mysterious stage of consciousness called turiya, i.e., the unmanifest state of Purusha.

30-32:1

Obstacles that may appear during sadhana and how to get past them.

1. Disease.

2. Lethargy.

3. Well-being.

4. Lack of action.

5. Laziness.

6. Strong desires.

7. Wrong perception.

8. Instability.

9. Shaking.

10. Pain.

11. Depression.

Knowing and being prepared is essential; difficulties and obstacles are part of the sadhana's path. When the consciousness is turned inwards, the metabolism and functions of the body change. You may fall asleep during meditation or have different perceptual experiences.

The person often does not care about their personal life, family, and other chores. You may experience doubts and feel unsure if the sadhana is correct or you will reach the goal.

You must focus on one principle – a mantra or a symbol to eliminate obstacles. One should, therefore, stick to a particular mantra or symbol and not change it. Otherwise, the obstacles will become a fact.

There is no real difference between the symbols, but if you change the symbol, confusion is created in the mind.

33:1

Creating Opposite Virtues – The Four Attitudes.

Maitrīkarunāmuditopeksānam sukhaduhkhapunyāpuṇyaviṣay-āṇām bhāvanātaśchittaprasādanam

Maitri: kindness, karuna: compassion, mudito: joy, upeksanam: indifference, sukha: happiness, duhkha: suffering, punya: virtue, apunya: burden, visayanam: goal, bhavanatah: attitude, chitta: mind, prasadanam: pure.

To concentrate the mind, it must first be purified and stilled. It is done by developing attitudes of kindness, compassion, joy, indifference, and respect for individuals and events that create happiness, suffering, virtues, or mistakes.

Through these attitudes, which are:

1. Friendship with the happy.
2. Compassion for the unfortunate.
3. Gratitude and joy for what goes well.
4. Indifference to what goes wrong.

It creates a calm and undisturbed mind. It is part of the nature of the mind to be drawn to the outside world. It is not part of the nature of the mind to look inward. When turning the mind inward, one must first remove obstacles and impurities. These four attitudes remove these obstacles on both a conscious and an unconscious level.

34:1

Control of prana.

Prachchhardanavidhāraṇābhyām vā prāṇasya

Prachchhardana: rechaka, vidharaan, bhyam: kumbakha, va: eller, pranasya; breathing.

By prolonging and keeping the spirit out, one can control the mind.

The whole mental structure consists of four different parts. Depending on the individual's temperament, different yoga paths fit differently.

1. Karma Yoga – dynamic people.

2. Bhakti yoga – emotional individuals.

3. Raya, Kriya, Swara yoga – psychic.

4. Jnana Yoga – intellectual persons.

We are often a mixture of all these and can benefit from practicing all paths. We should choose a sadhana that suits us best to create as little resistance as possible.

Patanjali describes pranayama and how we can calm our minds by keeping the spirit inside and out of the body through three locks. He describes maha bandha, where you do jalandhara, uddiyana, and moola bandha while keeping your breath out. If you are a beginner, you can practice rechaka and kapalbhati to begin with.

With the help of these exercises, the mind is calmed. It is said that the mind has two supports: prana and vasana. These are supports on which the mind rests, and the consciousness works. If you delete one of these, the other also disappears automatically.

Pranan can be both rough and subtle. The subtle pran exists in the form of energy, and the coarse pran is our breathing.

There are five main prana vayu that we have touched on before: prana, apana, udana, samana, and vyana vayu. There are also five smaller pranas: devatta, nada, kurma, krikara and dhananjaya. All of these control different parts of the body's functions:

Prana controls our inhalation and acts in the mouth and nose, digests food, separates nutrients from food, converts the water in the body into sweat and urine, and controls the secretion of the glands. Its area is between the heart and the nose.

The apana removes impurities and residues from the body and moves downward. Its area is around the navel and feet.

Samana works in our limbs and nadis. It acts in the area around the heart and navel.

Udana maintains our muscular strength and the energy that prevails when our karmic body leaves our physical body during death. It acts in the area around the neck and head.

Vyana controls blood circulation and moves through our nerves.

Nada controls coughing and sneezing, kurma controls contractions, krikara controls hunger and thirst, devatta creates drowsiness and sleep, and dhananjaya maintains nutrition.

There are also fine channels in the body called nadis. Prana / impulses and signals flow to and from the brain through these. In total, we have about seventy-two thousand different nadis.

Ida, pingala, and sushuman are the three most important nadis, of which sushumna is the most crucial channel for spiritual consciousness. These three start from the Mooladhara chakra and meet in the Ajna chakra.

Our breathing controls our thoughts in the present, past, and future. During the day, breathing alternates through the right and left nostrils. You usually breathe for one hour through the right nostril and then one hour through the left nostril and about twelve times a day through each. The left nostril is called the ida, and the right is the pingala. When the breathing changes from pingala to ida or from ida to pingala, the sushumna flows temporarily.

Performing heavy work is best suited when pingala nadi is flowing. When ida nadi flows, lighter work is best done. When sushumna nadi flows, meditation is best suited. We can control the flow through the nostrils with the help of various exercises.

35:1
Pay attention to sensory experiences.
Viṣayavatī vā pravṛttirutpannā manasah sthitinibandhanī
Visayavati: sensual, va: or, pravrttih: functioning, panning: arises, manasah: of the mind, sthiti: steadfastness, nibandhani: which binds.

The mind can be made steady by keeping it active with sensory experiences.

Suppose you experience Ishwara pranidhara, maha bandha, or pra-
nayama, which is challenging to practice. In that case, you can instead
use different sensory experiences such as sight, hearing, smell, taste,
and touch to create a steady and calm mind.

Nada yoga (antar mouna).
Trataka.
Kirtan.
Mantra.

36:1
Experience the inner light – optional meditation on what the mind is
drawn to naturally.
Viśokā vā jyotiṣmatī
Visoka: without sorrow, va: or, jyotismati: filled with light.

When filled with light, the state beyond grief can control the mind.

The mind can also be stilled by experiencing the inner calm and the
clear white light between the eyebrows – bhrumadhya or through
nada, concentration on sound. This inner glow is calm, still, and pea-
ceful and is experienced during deep meditation when you are sattvic,
and Kundalini Shakti flows through the sushumna and activates all
your chakras. The sound is spandam – aum, the sound of creation and
comsos; you hear it as a beeping sound of Bindu slowly increasing in
power. When you see the light and hear the sound, you are connected.
You send, and you receive the intensity of the cosmos. You are one with
the universe's intelligence, the collective consciousness – God.

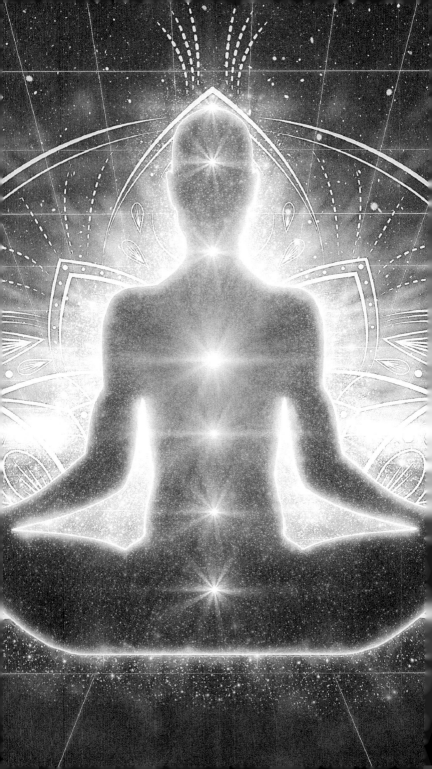

MEDITATION

Meditation aims to establish contact with his inner self and increase his self-awareness. The goal is to realize oneself. When a person achieves self-realization, they communicate with their innermost self and identify their existence – their life, based on their true self and not based on their ego. During meditation, one tries to establish an observed self, which means studying one's thoughts objectively and neutrally. Thus, gaining a perspective on one's thoughts, feelings, and existence is necessary.

The purpose of meditation is to explore the different regions of the mind, learn how the mind works, and train it to surpass the mind finally. In practical terms, meditation is about emptying the mind of thoughts by concentrating on the present through an activity or method.

ACTIVE MEDITATION

Active meditation means breathing with some form of movement to calm the thoughts and get into the present. Examples of active meditation are yoga, qigong, and tai chi. Dynamic meditation can also be part of our everyday life through walks, eating, etc. if you do it with the presence of putting your feet up and breathing. How it feels in the body, etc.

PASSIVE MEDITATION

Passive meditation – which most people may associate with meditation – means you are silent to practice some meditation techniques. One trains the mind through a specific method or process to put oneself in a meditative state.

Unlike in the past, research has recently begun to look at the holistic aspect of man a little more. Research on meditation has increased enormously. The reason for this may be the increased mental disorders and diseases that are today a public health problem in many countries. The current research that has been done on yoga and meditation shows clear and measurable results on stress-related issues such as neck and back problems, headaches, depression, anxiety, weight problems, and difficulty sleeping.

To overcome these mental problems, meditation has become an increasingly recommended and used method. More and more psychologists today advise their clients to practice meditation to connect with their inner self and emotions, for example. Psychology has now come to believe that the regular stage of a human being is a constant joy.

In research on meditation, pulsating electrical voltages are measured, which the brain gives rise to so-called brain waves. These brain waves are measured via EEG (Electro Encephalo Gram: electric-brain registration). These waves can display different frequencies, which are divided into four stages. The first stage is called beta waves and is the one we have during normal waking. Alpha waves are the second stage, and we are then relaxed and have a milder state of mind than meditation. We have theta waves when we dream.

Conversely, children may be in this stage when awake, but it is less common in adults. Delta waves are likened to deep sleep (without dreams). An experienced yogi can go from beta waves to delta waves during meditation. Research has also shown that those who have practiced meditation for a long time have more stable brain waves (have constant coherence) and a more excellent mental balance, i.e., triggers endorphins that strengthen the immune system.

Physiologically, meditation reduces muscle tension, improves respiratory rhythm, digestion, immune system, blood pressure, and heart rate, and increases the efficiency of the internal organs.

Many people who meditate regularly experience that they get more energy, become more alert, and sleep better; the stress level in the body decreases, concentration and the ability to focus are strengthened, and the ability to perform and oxygen uptake is improved.

The autonomic nervous system is divided into the sympathetic nervous system and the parasympathetic nervous system. The sympathetic nervous system is usually called the "fight or flight defense system," which is the system that is activated during mental or physical stress. When this is activated, the pupils dilate, blood pressure increases, digestion decreases, and blood sugar increases. The parasympathetic nervous system is the opposite, starting when the body is at rest. It lowers blood pressure, stimulates digestion, improves healing processes, and secretes oxytocin (the body's calm and growth hormone). These two systems complement each other.

Today's society and our lives result in the sympathetic nervous system being activated in many people almost all the time. The sympathetic nervous system is meant to be activated only for short periods. Still, as today's threats often consist of fears of being unable to pay bills, worries about the job, etc., they often become activated for longer. It leads to people always being tense, unhappy, and having a more challenging time resisting illness. If the sympathetic nervous system is activated, it can also lead to high blood pressure, diabetes, heart attack, and several mental disorders linked to stress.

The only way to prevent this is through physical and mental relaxation and, of course, with good sleep. Meditation provides both physical and psychological relaxation. We must also learn to react differently to our surroundings and what we are exposed to daily so that the adrenaline content only sometimes increases.

THINKING ABOUT MEDITATION

When sitting down for meditation, thinking about a few things is essential. The first preparation is that you can sit undisturbed, where you feel silent. Turn off all phones and make sure no one is disturbed. The morning or before bedtime are the best times for meditation. Also, remember not to eat too close to the meditation, as the body is full of digestion, and a lot of blood and energy is drawn in from the body to the stomach. Ensure you have done yoga or exercised before so that all restlessness is out of your body. Ensure your signal systems are balanced by asanas so that Kundalini Shakti can flow freely in the sushumna nadi and activate your chakras on the way up to the Sahasrara chakra.

Then, ensure you have something to sit on: a meditation pillow, a regular pillow, or a chair. Take the time to find a comfortable sitting position. It would help if you sat comfortably as you will sit still for a while. A popular sitting position is siddhasana, where you sit on the buttocks with the legs outstretched, insert one foot towards the groin, and place the other foot just in front of the shin or on top of the shin. Make sure you are sitting in a three-point position where both buttocks are in contact with the ground and both knees.

You place your hands on your knees with the palm facing down and let your thumb and forefinger meet in jnana mudra. Alternatively, place the proper back of the hand in the left palm and let the thumbs meet in bhairavi mudra. It is essential that you feel your hands resting securely so that you can relax your shoulders.

Feel that you are sitting with a straight spine where the weight from the upper body can fall straight down through the pelvis. Insert your chin slightly next to your chest so your neck can relax and close your eyes. Have a little weight forward on the pelvis so you do not collapse with your back.

Then start by landing in yourself with your thoughts and presence, calm the mind, and relax the body with kaya stahairyam. Then begin your chosen meditation technique with, for example, ajapa japa. It is essential not to have any expectations of the meditation and what one is believed to experience.

There are also various obstacles that one may encounter during meditation, such as thoughts and feelings. There can be obstacles such as anger, pride, and selfishness, which can be trained away, among other things. Practice yamas and niyamas. If any ideas or feelings arise during the meditation, become aware of them, see them, but then let them float on with the next exhalation and then return to focusing on the chosen meditation technique.

When the mind is still, and you are sattvic, the white light between the eyebrows – bhrumadhya, slowly emerges. Kundalini Shakti flows through the sushumna nadi, and all your chakras are activated. You hear a beeping sound from Bindu, which is gradually increasing power. When you see the light and hear the sound, you are connected.

*If it is difficult to calm down, it can be advantageous to have done so-
mething active before setting out for meditation, such as taking a walk
or doing a yoga session. It is also essential to have regularity in your
meditation practice.*

CLASSICAL TECHNIQUES FOR MEDITATION

*The classic sitting positions for meditation (meditation asanas) are
padmasana, siddhasana, siddha yoni asana, and swastikasana. For
beginners (and Westerners who are often stiff and have narrower hips),
you can also sit in sukhasana or ardha padmasana. You can do so if
you need to sit on a chair for various reasons. The principle is that the
sitting position should be comfortable and support the body during
meditation so you can relax. It's about something other than sitting
nicely. The back must be straight so that the prana can flow upwards in
the body. You can also lie comfortably on your back, but then there is
the risk of falling asleep.*

*Important mudras during meditation include jnana / chin mudra,
bhairavi mudra, and khechari mudra.*

JNANA MUDRA

*Place your hands on your knees with your palms facing down, and let
your thumb and forefinger meet.*

CHIN MUDRA

*Place your hands on your knees with the palm facing up, and let your
thumb and forefinger meet.*

BHAIRAVI MUDRA

*You place the proper back of the hand in the left palm and let your
thumbs meet.*

KHECHARI MUDRA
Roll up the tongue so that you place the back of the tongue up in the palate with gentle pressure.

UJJAYI PRANAYAMA
Ujjayi pranayama is also called the psychic / winning breath. Start by placing the back of the tongue up in the palate in the khechari mudra, narrow in the air passage, and strive for a whispering / hissing – "ah" sound. Breathe through your nose, but feel that the breathing and the sound come far in from the throat. It sounds like when you blow mist on a mirror with an open mouth. Children usually say that the sound is similar to Darth Vader's breathing in Star Wars.

Ujjayi pranayama is used in many different meditation techniques (and also during the practice of asanas) as it calms the nervous system and lowers blood pressure. It also emits a sound as a focal point to draw attention to. Breathing in this way also means that you retain the heat.

BHRUMADHYA
Bhrumadhya is a trigger point for the Ajna chakra (third eye). The word bhrumadhya means eyebrow center, also where this point is located.

CHIDAKASHA
Chidakasha can be explained as our inner mental television screen. It is visualized as space before our closed eyes, where our psychic event / event appears – "what the mind carries." Chidakasha stands for "area of knowledge," and Akasha means space—our microcosmos.

JAPA YOGA

Using the mantra, Japa yoga is an effective technique for returning the mind to the present. Japa means repetition of a mantra. The mantra affects us physically and mentally with the help of the word's meaning and vibrations within one. Mantra meditation cleanses the subconscious mind and causes the thought activity to decrease, as the mind does not receive any new stimulus. It makes it easier to get in touch with your inner self.

Constantly repeating the mantra makes the mind concentrated and relaxed and gives us inner peace. It is important not to force focus on the mantra but to let it come naturally from within. One can practice japa with different forms of mantras; it can be mantras that one pronounces aloud (baikhari), mantras to whisper (upanshu), mental mantras (mansaik), or written mantras (likhit). You often recite the mantra a certain number of times, and to help you with the count, you can have a mala, a rosary with pearls. You can practice Japa yoga while sitting in a meditation position and performing other daily activities. If you are rajasic, you should be careful not to increase the tempo of the mantra or become stressed by it.

AJAPA JAPA

Ajapa japa is a complete sadhana (spiritual practice where one eventually achieves self-realization). By regularly practicing ajapa japa for a long time, subconscious desires and fears will finally come to the

surface, which one will then view with a witness attitude and thus get to the root of physical and mental problems and can change them.

Japa means repetition of a mantra. Ajapa japa means constant awa-

reness. Traditionally, the mantra So-Ham is used, but it is possible to use any mantra if, for example, you have received a mantra from your guru.

HARI OM TAT SAT

A guided meditation often ends with Hari Om Tat Sat in classical yoga.

Hari Om and Tat Sat are two different mantras brought together; Hari Om is one, and Tat Sat is the other. Hari stands for the manifested universe and life, the energy – Shakti. Om stands for the absolute reality, the consciousness – Shiva. Reality consists of the complete (incomprehensible) and the obvious / the more concrete. This reality is presented in the mantra Hari Om Tat Sat. Satya means truth. Tat Sat means "it is the truth." Hari Om Tat Sat means both the concrete – what I can see and the unknown or incomprehensible, which is also part of the same reality and not different.

YOGASCHITTA VRITTI NIRODHAH

(When the movements of the mind are still, yoga occurs)

KUNDALINI YOGA

ALL ABOUT OUR CHAKRA!

KUNDALINI YOGA

WHAT IS KUNDALINI?

Kundalini is the stagnant energy that exists in every human being. It sits at the bottom of the spine in the perineum or pelvic floor (between the urine and the excretory organs) in men and at the cervix (the base of the cervix in women). Here, you will find Mooladhara chakra.

With the help of yogic techniques such as asana, pranayama, Kriya yoga, and meditation, one can increase the flow of prana in the body and direct it down to Mooladhara chakra to awaken the Kundalini Shakti. When the Kundalini energy begins to rise upwards along the Sushumna Nadi and through the chakras, the dormant parts of the brain that are in contact with the respective chakras awaken. This process allows us to access our brain's capacity and raise consciousness.

The awakening of Kundalini should slowly be done and systematically. The body and mind should be prepared slowly. This way, you avoid any risks that a rise may entail. One should not try to control or influence the mind as such. The mind is an "extension" of the body, and therefore, it is easiest to start with the body and gradually move on with prana, nadis, and chakras.

HOW THE KUNDALINI WAS DISCOVERED

Since the beginning, man has been involved in and experienced events of a supernatural nature. When it so happened that one would feel what others were thinking and wanting, the inner visions manifested, and dreams came true. It was noticed that a particular crowd had an

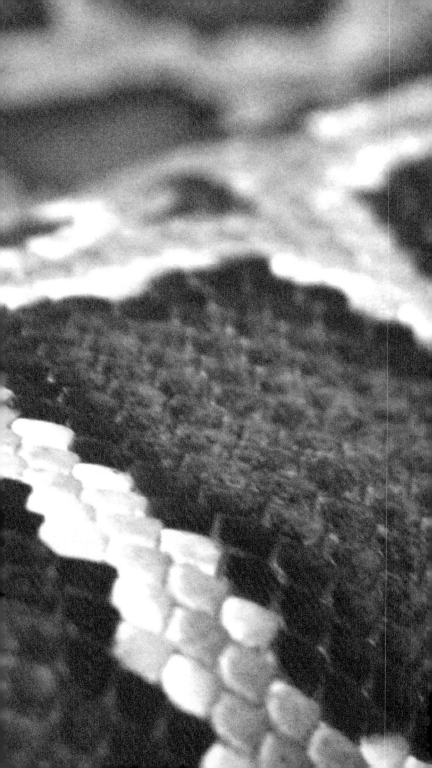

extraordinary ability to express their creativity through art, music, and poetry. Some people had a strong drive and zest for life, while others barely managed to get up in the morning. Man became curious as to what was the cause of these differences. In the end, through one's own experience, one could conclude that man had a unique form of energy. In some, this energy was dormant, in development in others, and fully awakened in very few. This energy was called after gods and deities. After they also discovered prana, they started calling it prana Shakti. In tantrism, this energy is called Kundalini Shakti.

DIFFERENT NAMES

In Sanskrit, Kundalini means "spiral" or "something that is rolled up." Kundalini Shakti has thus traditionally been described as something that has just been rolled up. Nevertheless, the meaning of the whole thing has often needed to be understood. Kundalini derives from the word – kunda, which refers to "a more profound place" or a pit. Kundalini refers to Shakti, or the power, energy in its dormant state. When it wakes up and manifests itself, it is called Devi, Kali, Durga, Saraswati, Lakshmi, or something else, depending on the characteristics and qualities it evokes in man.

In Christianity, terms such as "the path of the initiated" or "the stairs to heaven" are used. These refer to the Kundalini that rises along the sushumna nadi. The Christian cross symbolizes Kundalini rising and the resulting spiritual beauty. In all spiritual paths, whether one is talking about samadhi, nirvana, moksha, unity, kaivalya, or liberation, it is the Kundalini awakening one is referring to.

KUNDALINI, DURGA, KALI

When you can positively handle a raised Kundalini, its quality is called

Durga. If Kundalini instead wakes up when you are still unprepared and not ready to take it, it is called Kali.

The goddess Kali is illustrated as naked black and wears a rosary of one hundred and eight human skulls representing memories from previous lives. Her blood-red outstretched tongue symbolizes raja guna, whose circular movement pattern powers all creative activity. She wants to urge Sadhakas to take control of raja guna.

Durga is a beautiful goddess who is illustrated riding a tiger. She has eight arms that represent the eightfold elements. She wears a rosary with fifty-two human skulls that symbolize her wisdom, power, and the fifty-two letters of the Sanskrit alphabet. Durga eliminates all the evil consequences that life can carry and comes with strength and peace. This force is released from Mooladhara chakra.

KUNDALINI PHYSIOLOGY

When Kundalini begins to rise, it passes different phases on its way up to the cosmic consciousness – Shiva, where they finally merge. The highest consciousness – Shiva, has its seat in Sahasrara chakra – the super consciousness, at the top of the head. This seat is called Hiranyagarbha – the womb of consciousness in the Vedic texts and Tantrism. It is connected to the pituitary gland. Just below is another psychic center called the Ajna chakra, connected to the pineal gland, the seat of intuitive consciousness. It is located at the top of the spine and the height of the eyebrow center – bhrumadhya. Ajna chakra is essential as it is connected to the Mooladhara and Sahasrara chakra.

Chakras are energy vortices that are experienced to vibrate and rotate at different speeds. There are thousands of chakras in the human body.

In tantra and yoga, only a few are used for filling the entire spectrum of human evolution and life – physically and mentally, from the rough to the polished. Six chakras have a direct connection to the dormant parts of the brain.

Through nadis, energy flows to and from the chakras. Nadis are channels where prana (vital) and mana (mental) energy flows through and out to all parts of the body. There are about seventy-two thousand nadis. Three of these are extra important as they control the flow of prana and the consciousness of all other nadis. These are ida, pingala, and sushumna. Ida controls all the mental activity, and pingala controls all the vital activity. Ida is known as the moon, and pingala as the sun. Sushumna is the channel for the flow of spiritual consciousness. Ida and pingala do not flow in the body simultaneously but alternate. When the left nostril is open, ida nadi flows; when the right nostril is available, the pingala flows. When the pingala flows, the left part of the brain is active, and when the ida flows, the right part is active. In this way, nadis control our brain, way of acting, and consciousness.

Suppose you can get prana and chitta, ie. ida and pingala flow simultaneously; you can get both halves of the brain to cooperate in thinking and action. This does not happen in our everyday daily lives. For this to happen, it is required that the sushumna is in contact with Kundalini Shakti.

Sushumna nadi is like a hollow tube with three more tubes in it. One is more subtle than the other. These tubes, or nadis, are called sushumna (denotes tamas), vajrini (denotes rajas), chitrini (denotes sattva) and Brahma (represents consciousness). The highest consciousness born of Kundalini Shakti passes through Brahma.

When Kundalini wakes up, the sushumna passes up to the Ajna chakra. Mooladhara chakra acts as a powerful engine. To start this engine, pranic energy is needed, and it is created with the help of pranayamas. The prana is then directed downwards in the body to the Mooladhara chakra. From there, it is then directed upwards towards the Ajna chakra. If the sushumna nadi is not open, the energy cannot be distributed, which means that the prana remains in the Mooladhara chakra.

Ida and pingala nadi are constantly flowing, but their power is weak. It is only when the sushumna is awakened that enlightenment can take place. Kundalini yoga is based on reviving the sushumna; when awakened, contact between the highest and lowest levels of consciousness is enabled. Then Kundalini can wake up and rise from Mooladhara up along the Sushumna and become one with Shiva in Sahasrara.

THE MYSTICAL TREE

In the Bhagavad Gita, you can read about the immortal tree that grows up and down, with the roots up and the leaves and branches down. It is said that he who knows the tree also knows the truth of life. This tree is found in the human body and nervous system. The tree leaves symbolize thoughts, feelings, obstacles, etc. The roots and the spine of the trunk represent the brain. You have to climb from the top of the tree (in this case, from the root) and up to the roots. In Kabbalah, this tree is called the "tree of life." In the Bible, it is called the "Tree of Knowledge." Anyone who tries to move upwards from Mooladhara chakra to Sahasrara chakra thus climbs to the roots.

KUNDALINI AND OUR BRAIN

Humans often use only a tenth of the brain's total capacity. This small part stores our knowledge of what we think and do. The rest is known as the dormant and inactive part of the brain. It is passive because the energy is not enough to keep it awake. The active part of the brain gets its power from ida and pingala nadi, while the dormant portion only has access to pingala, i.e., prana, or life energy. It lacks conscious energy, i.e., ida or manas.

To awaken the sleeping part of the brain, we must charge the front part of the brain with prana and consciousness. We must also awaken sushumna nadi. We do this by practicing pranayamas regularly for an extended period. With the help of Kundalini yoga, one could discover that the different parts of the brain are connected to our chakras. To access dormant parts of the brain, one must work on awakening the chakras in the body. Chakras can be described as switches.

In the same way, the Mooladhara chakra is used as a "switch" to awaken Kundalini, which has its seat in Sahasrara, but most of us find it easier to get in touch with Mooladhara chakra. Each chakra works individually. This means that if Kundalini wakes up in Mooladhara, it goes straight up to Sahasrara. Or, if it wakes up in Swadhisthana, it also goes from there straight up to Sahasrara. Kundalini can be awakened in a chakra or collectively in all chakras simultaneously. When Kundalini awakens in an individual chakra, the consciousness is filled with what is characteristic of that particular chakra.

WHAT KUNDALINI SHAKTI IS
There are many different descriptions of what Kundalini Shakti is. Many yogis believe that Kundalini Shakti is pranic energy that flows through the Sushumna associated with the spine. They believe that Kundalini is part of the pranic flow in our energy body and that there is no physical / anatomical equivalent.

Other yogis experience Kundalini as part of the signals that flow along the nerve pathways and travel along the spinal cord up to specific brain parts. However, most agree that Kundalini's psychophysiological experience manifests in the spine.

METHODS FOR AWAKENING:

In Tantrism, various techniques are used to awaken Kundalini Shakti. These can be practiced individually or in combination with each other.

AWAKENED IN CONNECTION WITH BIRTH

A few children are born with an already awake Kundalini. These children look at life very clearly and have a highly developed way of thinking and a very unusual way of looking at life. They often have no normal social relationship with their parents because they see them as "those who gave them life."

MANTRA

It is a powerful, gentle, and risk-free method. However, it requires patience, time, discipline, and regularity. Through mantra repetition and the vibration of sound, a wave of patterns is created that affects the mind. The physical, mental, and emotional body is cleansed. It is essential to focus the mantra on something by, for example, focusing on the tip of the nose or a chakra.

TAPASYA

It is a psychological procedure where you start a process that, from the root, eliminates terrible habits that have created weakness and hindered development and willpower. Willpower is the core of tapasya. To enable growth and willpower, you want to curb the inner fire, live in celibacy, say no to lust, be restrained, and deny your desires.

ASUHADHI – using herbs

This is the fastest and most effective method besides tantric initiation. It should not be confused with the use of drugs. Asuhadhi is a risky method that should only be done under the guidance of a guru.

PSYCHEDELIA – with the help of psychoactive drugs

Ayahuasca, LSD, DMT, magic mushrooms, etc., are all psychoactive drugs used to expand the mind and to awaken Kundalini Shakti quickly. Shamans have been using mind-expanding drugs since ancient times. There are significant risks associated with developing the mind using drugs. Psychoses, delusions, and other unpleasant mental experiences can be triggered, even if they do not create a physical dependence. Awakening Kundalini Shakti too quickly and powerfully without being prepared is possible. Be cautious. Take it slow.

RAJA YOGA

With Raja yoga, one merges the individual consciousness with the universal superconscious. This is done step by step with the help of concentration, meditation, and the experience of unity with the absolute and highest self. When you focus and calm your mind, the sushumna opens, enabling Kundalini's rising. This mild method is experienced as problematic by many because it requires a lot of patience and discipline.

PRANAYAMA

Pranayamas are very powerful. Kundalini can be awakened very quickly if you are well prepared, live healthy, and have a calm and safe place to practice breathing exercises. Pranayamas strongly affect the body, creating heat while lowering the temperature in the inner body. Breathing changes the pattern of brain waves. It is essential to cleanse the body with the help of shatkarmas before entering the process to handle the rapid changes better. Breathing is the link between Hatha and Kundalini yoga.

KRIYA YOGA

This is the simplest method for people living in the modern world. Here, you do not have to confront the mind like, e.g., Raja yoga. People who are Sattvic may find it easy to awaken Kundalini through Raja yoga. Still, if you have a tumultuous mind that is constantly in motion, it only creates even more tension, guilt, complexity, and sometimes even schizophrenia. When practicing Kriya yoga, Kundalini Shakti is awakened slowly and methodically.

TANTRIC INITIATION

This method requires an understanding of what Shiva and Shakti stand for. You have to change your approach to passions and desires in life. Under the guidance of a guru, this is the fastest way to Kundalini awakening.

SHAKTIPAT

A guru performs this method. One experiences a temporary state of awakening – samadhi.

SURRENDER YOURSELF

This path means that one does not strive to awaken Kundalini Shakti. You let it happen when it happens and if it happens. It is believed that a strong enough will can arouse Kundalini.

PREPARATIONS

It is essential to learn Kundalini yoga from a competent teacher so that one knows for sure that the process is going the right way. It is also necessary to be physically, mentally, and emotionally prepared. Waking up Kundalini Shakti can take time; you can count on it being a long process. However, nothing says that Kundalini cannot wake up quickly. What takes time is learning to keep the Kundalini alive.

The Sushumna must be open; otherwise, Kundalini will rise along the ida or pingala, leading to complications. The elements, chakras, and nadis must also be purified for Kundalini to flow freely. This is done with the help of asanas, pranayamas and Hatha yoga shatkarmas.

Surya namaskar and surya bheda pranayama cleanses pingala nadi. Shatkarmas and pranayamas open up the sushumna. You start by cleaning the elements with shatkarmas. Then continue with asanas and pranayamas. After that, you can continue with mudras and bandhas. Then, you are ready to start with Kriya yoga.

KARMA YOGA

Karma yoga is an essential part of spiritual development. Without Karma yoga, evolution will stop no matter what method one follows. Karma yoga prepares the mind. Positive and negative partners become visible, consciousness is broadened, and concentration is strengthened. Karma yoga is not a direct cause of Kundalini awakening but an essential part of the process.

DIFFERENT AWAKENINGS

It is crucial to distinguish between the awakening of Kundalini, chakras, and sushumna nadi. It should also be possible to differentiate between an awakening between Mooladhara and Kundalini. The first step in awakening Kundalini Shakti is to create harmony between ida and pingala nadi. The next step is to awaken the chakra system, which *leads to the sushumna opening and allows the Kundalini Shakti to wake up.*

You do not have to worry about negative consequences when the process occurs in this order. If Kundalini instead wakes up before the sushumna is open, the energy will remain in the Mooladhara chakra and create sexual and neurotic disorders. Should any chakra not be available, Kundalini will get stuck in its path and create stagnation in development.

Harmony between ida and pingala nadi:

Pingala stands for vital energy in the body. Ida stands for conscious energy. These two nadis control the brain's two hemispheres, which in turn control all activity in the body. It is not the awakening of these two that one strives for but the synchronization between them. As is well known, these control the body's temperature, digestion, hormonal secretion, brain waves, and the whole body's system. Lousy food and lifestyle disturbs and creates an imbalance between them, which leads to physical and mental illness. Sushumna can only wake up when ida and pingala flow in harmony. Hatha, pranayamas, and Raja yoga are the best methods to balance ida and pingala—especially nadi shodhana.

Awaken the chakras:

All chakras must be balanced before the sushumna can wake up. Every little part of the body is connected to a chakra. Asanas open up the chakras in a gentle way. Sometimes, a chakra can open quickly. Then feelings of fear, anxiety, passion, depression, etc., can emerge that have connections to previous experiences from previous lives.

Awaken the sushumna:

It takes a lot of patience to awaken the sushumna nadi. You can expect to have experiences of a more intense nature than those that come when a chakra is awakened. These experiences are often entirely illogical and strange. Hatha yoga and pranayamas are essential for awakening sushumna nadi.

KUNDALINI SINKS IN

After a rise, Kundalini will fall again. But the mind and consciousness will still be affected and changed. You get a higher state of consciousness. Our whole lives and thoughts are concerned—emotions, body, and mind. Kundalini will be what characterizes life.

When Shiva and Shakti become one in Sahasrara chakra, one experiences samadhi, and silent parts of the brain wake up. In this state, one is entirely unaware of opposites, man and woman, Shiva and Shakti – everything is the same. During the experience of samadhi, Bindu develops. Bindu means point and encompasses the entire cosmos. It is the seat of human intelligence and all creation. After a while, the Bindu is divided into two, and the duality of Shiva and Shakti becomes a reality again.

Samadhi can be likened to the condition of an infant. One does not know the difference between a man and a woman, and there is no physical or sexual difference. They separate when Shiva and Shakti return to the rough plane, down to the Mooladhara chakra. Duality exists in the mind in the world that consists of name and form but not in samadhi.

When Kundalini sinks, and you return to physical reality, you do it with a changed consciousness. You may live with the same patterns, desires, and passions. What makes the difference is that you observe life as if it were a spectacle.

You are in the theater of life as before but as a spectator. The changed consciousness is manifested through one. You are in contact with the parts of the brain that were previously silent. One is in contact with the universe's knowledge, power, and wisdom.

THE EXPERIENCE OF THE AWAKENING

A Kundalini rise can be likened to an explosion that takes you from one plane of consciousness to another plane of being. You travel through the borderland where perceptions, feelings, and experiences change character. It is a journey between what you have experienced and the inexperienced.

The awakening takes place step by step and can take time. The preliminary awakening, usually the first step, is the experience of light at bhrumadhya. This usually develops over a long period in a very mild way and rarely creates any negative experiences. After a while, your appetite and need for sleep may decrease, and your mind is still. When the Kundalini rise finally takes place, it happens with power, and sometimes, you can experience things that are difficult to comprehend. One of the most common experiences is feeling "a current" along the spine. One can experience a burning sensation in Mooladhara and an energy flowing up and down along the Sushumna. You can also hear sounds in the form of drums, bells, music, birds, and flutes. You can also experience anger, passion, and other repressed emotions that emerge. This usually passes within a few days. Some develop siddhis, which after a while also disappear.

You can lose your appetite for weeks, become depressed, lose interest in life, and experience everything as very sad at the same time as the mind can become very mobile and creative. You might start writing poetry, creating music, or some other art. This flattens out after a while, and you land again in your everyday and ordinary lives. From the outside, everything looks like before, but you have an increased inner awareness and ability to observe. Headaches and insomnia can occur in some people when Kundalini wakes up.

It is easy to confuse the awakening of our chakras, nadis, and sushumna with a Kundalini rise. When the chakra is opened, you get experiences that are usually pleasant and satisfying. They are rarely nasty or scary. When you get enjoyable experiences during meditation or the kirtan or can feel the presence of your guru, it is a chakra awakening that takes place, not Kundalini.

When sushumna wakes up, you can experience the spine shining or a streak of light. You can also have sensual experiences that can seem very confusing and illogical. You can smell, hear screams or cry, feel warm, or experience pain. Sometimes, you can get disease symptoms and fever that doctors can not diagnose. When Sushumna wakes up, you go through a form of depression, anorexia, and loneliness. You begin to understand your inner being, your true nature. Materia is experienced as nothing, and the body feels as if it were made of air, or you can feel as if you are not a part of the body. You can communicate with your surroundings, trees, animals, and water. You can start to anticipate things, but usually only boredom, accidents, and disasters. You can feel reluctant to do work, and it is good if, at this stage, you can be close to your guru to explain what is happening.

*Fine visions and experiences are not always a sushumna or Kundalini
awakening. It can still be chakras that open up or experiences of samskaras and archetypes that emerge due to the sadhana that one follows.
But to sum it up, a Kundalini awakening always creates more abilities,
siddhis. If you slowly begin to understand language better, you suddenly start to understand complicated things, become good at cooking,
get a hearing in music, etc. A gradual Kundalini awakening is taking
place. If you experience temporary sensations and powerful light phenomena or visions, other things may be connected to your chakras.*

DIET

*When Kundalini is awakened, it is essential to follow a proper diet
as the food affects the mind and human nature. During awakening,
physical changes occur in the body, mainly in the digestive system. The
body's internal temperature drops drastically, much lower than the
outer body temperature. Metabolism is slow, and oxygen consumption
decreases. The food must, therefore, be easy to break down.*

*The best is cooked food. Crushed wheat, barley, lentils, and dal are
preferred, preferably in liquid form. Fatty and heavy foods should be
avoided, and the amount of protein should be kept to a minimum, as
they strain the liver and require a lot of energy to break down. When
the mind changes, the liver works hard. It is good to increase the
carbohydrates in the diet, such as rice, potatoes, wheat, and corn. These
cause the internal body temperature to grow and do not require much
energy to digest.*

*Spices play a vital role in a Kundalini yogi. Coriander, cumin, anise,
black pepper, green pepper, cayenne, mustard seeds, cardamom, cinna-
mon, etc. support digestion. They store vital energy and keep the
internal body temperature.*

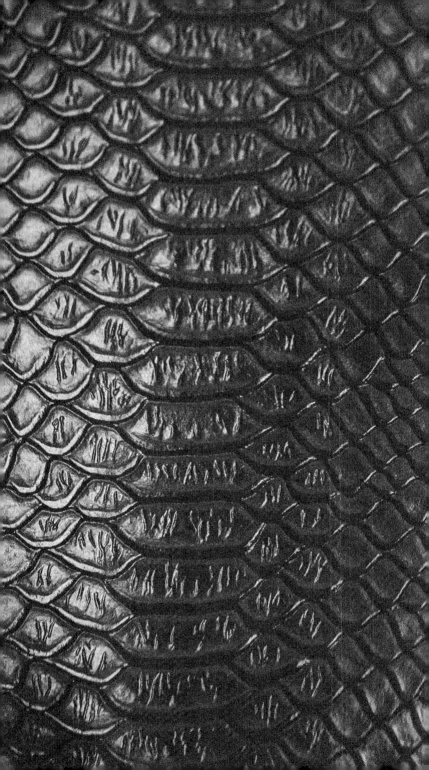

KRIYA YOGA

Awakening Kundalini is complex. Most yogic and religious paths are based on many rules that require incredible self-discipline. In the tantric tradition, Rishis developed a series of exercises that would be easy to follow and apply regardless of lifestyle, beliefs, or desires. Kriya yoga is one of the most potent tantric exercises and the path most suitable for the modern man. Kriya yoga aims to open the chakra system, purify the nadis, and awaken the Kundalini Shakti. Through the various kriyas, Kundalini is aroused gradually. It does not rise suddenly, which would be too difficult to handle.

Unlike other religions and yogic paths that often require robust mind control, one should not worry about the mind in Kriya yoga. Even if you can not concentrate or calm your mind, it does not matter – you develop anyway. Rishis in Kriya yoga believe that control of the mind is not necessary.

It is not always the mind's fault that it is anxious or restless. Hormones, indigestion, and a weak energy flow in the nervous system can be the cause. One should never blame the mind when it is disturbed, not even oneself. You are not stupid, wrong, unclean, or horrible, even if you think evil thoughts. Everyone suffers from these, even the most peaceful and devoted. Trying to push back from the mind and ideas and then see them come back again creates a division and, in the worst case, causes mental illness. There is no good or evil mind. They are both the same. The mind is nothing but energy. Anger, passion, gratitude, and joy are all different forms of the same energy. In Kriya yoga, one tries to utilize this energy without trying to silence or dampen it.

In Kriya yoga, one does not try to concentrate or meditate. Mental

147

control is not the purpose. The mind should flow freely and naturally. Kriya yoga is designed for individuals who struggle to sit still and stay focused for a long time. But – everyone should, whether you are tamasic, rajasic, or sattvic, practice Hatha yoga as a preparation. A tamasic person needs Hatha yoga to awaken the mind and body. A rajasic person needs Hatha yoga to balance the vital and mental energies in the body and mind. A sattvic person needs Hatha yoga to make it easier to awaken Kundalini. In other words, Hatha yoga is for everyone and is a preparation for Kriya yoga. You are usually ready for Kriya yoga if you have regularly practiced asanas, pranayamas, mudras, and bandhas for two years.

There are many Kriyas, but twenty are the most important and influential. These twenty are divided into two groups. The first nine are done with open eyes, and the remaining eleven are done with closed eyes.

In the first group of exercises, you mustn't close your eyes even if you feel very relaxed and have an easy time turning your mind inward. You can blink, rest, and take a break, but do not close your eyes.

The first Kriya is called Vipareeta Karani mudra. It is a method of creating a reverse process in the body. In Hatha Yoga Pradipika and the old tantric texts, you can read about this process:

"This nectar originates from the moon. As the sun consumes this nectar, the yogi ages. His body collapses, and dies. Through regular practice, the yogi should try to reverse this process. The nectar flowing from the moon (Bindu) towards the sun (Manipura) should be returned to the higher centers. When the flow of Amrit or nectar can be

*reversed, the sun will not consume it. The body will instead assimilate
it."*

*When the body has been cleansed with Hatha yoga, pranayamas, and
a pure diet, the nectar of the body is assimilated, and one experiences a
higher mental state. The mind is still, and you see and hear everything
much more straightforward.*

*It is said that one can influence and control the structure and energy
of the body and thus evoke peace, dharana, dhyana, or samadhi. The
various exercises in Kriya yoga, such as Vipareeta Karani mudra,
Amrit Pan, Khechari mudra, Moola bandha, Maha mudra, and Maha
Bheda mudra, regulate the nervous system. The prana in the body is
harmonized and balanced. You achieve a state of peace and tranquility
without having to fight against the mind. All this is done by creating
a flow of unused and natural chemicals in the body. Amrit is one of
them, and through Khechari mudra, you can make it flow.*

*Khechari mudra is a simple but essential technique used in most
kriyas. Turning the tongue upwards in the palate towards the nasal
passage stimulates specific glands and bandages, resulting in the Amrit
starting to flow—one experiences shoonyata, a state of nothingness, being, and awareness of everything. Body temperature drops, and alpha
waves begin to prevail. The mind is completely still.*

*When you have practiced yoga for a while and have reached the point
where you have achieved concentration and a complete inner stillness
in body, mind, and soul but still feel that there is more to discover, you
are ready for Kriya yoga. A calm mind, relaxed body, and proper understanding result from a spiritual life; however, it is not the ultimate*

goal. The deeper meaning of yoga is to change the experience's character, the mind's pattern, and its perception. Man's purpose in practicing yoga has been to expand the mind and release energy. It is tantra and the ultimate goal of Kriya yoga.

THE CHAKRA SYSTEM

In tantra and yoga, the lotus flower is used as a symbol for chakras. Man's spiritual development consists of three essential phases: ignorance, striving, longing, and enlightenment. In the same way, the lotus flower grows through three phases: clay, water, and air. It grows in mud (ignorance), grows up through the water to the surface (striving and longing), and finally, it comes up from the water and reaches the air and sunlight (enlightenment).

Each chakra is described as a lotus flower with a specific color and several petals. Each chakra consists of six different aspects:

1. Color.
2. Number of petals.
3. Yantra (geometric shape).
4. Beeja mantra (sound/vibration).
5. Animal symbol (represents previous stages of evolution).
6. Higher / eternal being (represents the higher consciousness).

OUR CHAKRAS
Our body has many chakras, but the most important ones are along our spine. There are also hidden so-called "Secret chakras." The eight most important chakras in our body are:

MOOLADHARA CHAKRA
The root chakra is located at the base of the spine and is the chakra that vibrates with the lowest frequency, i.e., the slowest of our seven chakras. Due to its frequency, its color is dark red, and has four petals.

The element associated with this chakra is earth and stands for the most physical and down-to-earth with us.

SWADHISTHANA CHAKRA

The Swadhisthana chakra is about two centimeters above the tailbone and is the center of our sexuality and reproductive ability. It has six petals, orange, and its element is water.

MANIPURA CHAKRA

The Manipura chakra is located at the spine at the solar plexus level. It has ten petals, and the color is yellow. Fire controls Manipura and is associated with will, worldly pursuit, ambition, and career.

ANAHATA CHAKRA

The Anahata chakra is located in the spine behind the heart. It has twelve petals, and the color is blue or green, depending on your yoga tradition. The element air dominates the chakra and controls our emotions and relationships with others. The Anahata chakra is also a symbol of love.

VISHUDDHI CHAKRA

Vishuddhi chakra is located in the neck and has sixteen petals. The color is violet, and the element is space (ether). It controls our communication with the environment on different levels.

AJNA CHAKRA

The Ajna chakra is located in the middle of the head at the pineal gland, and its contact area is the eyebrow center. It controls our paranormal abilities and siddhis. She is also called guru chakra or third eye. It is white and has two petals. It is associated with the mind, reason, intelligence, and intuition.

BINDU VISARGA

*According to tantra, Bindu visarga is located on the back of the head,
where the Brahmins usually have their tuft of hair. It represents the
crescent with a white drop, representing the manifestation of creation,
such as consciousness.*

SAHASRARA CHAKRA

*The chakra is located just above the head and is purple / red. It has a
thousand petals and represents pure consciousness. When Kundalini
Shakti reaches the Sahasrara chakra, we become enlightened, and
according to yoga, we enter nirvikalpa samadhi.*

KSHETRAM

*The exercises in Kundalini yoga usually focus on the trigger point of
the chakra, which has its place at the spine. It can be challenging to
experience initially, and many find it easier to focus on the point of
contact on the front of the body called the chakra kshetram. When
we focus on a kshetram, a sensation is created, passing via the nerve
pathways to the chakra and, from there, up to the brain. Mooladhara
has no contact point or kshetram.*

GRANTHIS

*We have three granthis (mental knots) in our physical body that are
obstacles to Kundalini. These are called Brahma, Vishnu, and Rudra.
They describe the strength of the Maya, the ignorance, and the attraction to material things—the level of consciousness. As an aspirant, one
must overcome these obstacles for Kundalini to flow unhindered.*

*Brahma granthi is in the Mooladhara chakra and is associated with
the desire for material things, physical satisfaction, and selfishness. It is
also responsible for tamas – negativity, lethargy, and ignorance.*

Vishnu granthi has its place in the Anahata chakra and is associated with emotional desires, depending on people and inner mental visions. It is linked to rajas and has tendencies toward passion, ambition, and determination.

Rudra granthi rules over the Ajna chakra. It is associated with the desire for siddhis, mental phenomena, and the image of ourselves as individuals.

THE EVOLUTION THROUGH THE CHAKRANA

Human evolution as individuals and as a race is a journey through our chakras. Mooladhara is the base, and Sahasrara is the very goal or end of evolution.

In animals, Mooladhara is the highest chakra. It is their Sahasrara. Until Mooladhara, evolution takes place by itself and is controlled by nature. When Kundalini reaches Mooladhara, development no longer happens automatically. Man is no longer subordinate to the laws of nature. Man is aware of time and space. Man has an ego; he can think, is aware that he is thinking, and knows that he is aware that he is thinking. Without the ego, there is no double consciousness. Animals do not have a double consciousness. Thus, man has a higher consciousness and must work to develop it. Therefore, it is said that Kundalini lies dormant in Mooladhara until it is awakened for further development.

Awakening Kundalini is a process. It may wake up to return to Mooladhara several times. When it finally reaches the Manipura chakra in a steady state, it will not turn again. What can happen is that it can get stuck in a chakra if there are blockages or if the sushumna is not open. Kundalini can remain in a chakra for several years or even a lifetime.

Before starting to practice Kundalini yoga, finding out which chakra Kundalini is located is essential. The easiest way to do this is to focus on each chakra individually for fifteen minutes over fifteen days. You will notice which chakra is most accessible to experience and stay focused on. Here is Kundalini Shakti.

Awakening our chakras plays a vital role in human evolution. It has nothing to do with mystery or anything occult. When the chakras are awakened, our consciousness and our mind change. This affects our daily lives as our mind controls how we act in different situations, relationships, and emotions.

Today, many children are born with open chakras and Kundalini. When these children grow up, they behave differently. Our modern society often sees these differences as something abnormal, and the result is often mental health care or similar. Going through conflicts within family and work is a common phenomenon. Still, when the mind and consciousness expand, one becomes extremely sensitive to everything in the mind: family, colleagues, and society. You can not overlook something that happens in life. Most people do not see it as usual, but it is a natural consequence of the awakened chakra. Consciousness becomes very receptive when the frequency of the mind changes.

Love, devotion, charity, etc., are all expressions of a mind affected by the chakra in balance. This is why so much emphasis is placed on awakening the Anahata chakra, or the heart chakra. All chakras are, of course, essential to open up, and all have different qualities. Still, you can see that most ancient scriptures emphasized awakening the Anahata, Ajna, and Mooladhara chakra. When Anahata is aroused, we get a deeper relationship with our family and all individuals.

When the chakras are opened, the mind changes automatically. Values change, and love and relationships change character. Disappointments and feelings of frustration are balanced, which leads to a better attitude toward ourselves and life.

PREPARATIONS FOR KRIYA YOGA

Kriya yoga is considered by many to be the most effective method of developing human consciousness. These exercises are said to be those that Shiva gave to his wife, Parvati. Kriyas are relatively simple and must be more potent for the average person to perform.

Before you start practicing Kriya yoga, it is essential that you can feel the chakras in the body, both mentally and physically, and be able to locate its kshetram. One should also know two mental passages in the body, "arohan" and "awarohan."

To develop in Kundalini yoga and preparation for Kriya yoga, it is essential to be well acquainted with the following techniques:

Vipareeta Karani asana
Ujjayi pranayama
Siddhasana / Siddha yoni asana
Unmani mudra
Khechari mudra
Ajapa Japa
Utthanpadasana
Shambhavi mudra
Moola bandha
Nasikagra drishti
Uddiyana bandha

Jalandhara bandha
Bhadrasana
Padmasana
Shanmuki mudra
Varjoli / Sahajoli mudra

IDA AND PINGALA

Yogis have described that man has three leading energy flows in the body. Ida, pingala and sushumna nadi. These can be roughly translated as mind, body, and spirit. Sushumna results from a balanced and harmonious flow between ida and pingala.

Nadis are flows of energy that move throughout our bodies. All the thousands of nadis that flow in the body are connected to the ida and pingala nadi that move along the spine. Every cell in our body, organ, brain, and mind is linked on a mental and physical level, which allows us to speak, think, and act in a balanced and correct way. Ida and pingala nadi are the ones who control the balance between them. By affecting a part of the system, the whole system is affected. This is how asanas, pranayamas, meditation, and the complete yogic system work. Yoga thus affects the entire system of nadis in our body.

Yogis and scientists have come to the same result, albeit with different ways of describing it. Man has two main modes through which he functions. The pattern of the brain is based on ida and pingala nadi, consciousness or knowledge, action or physical energy. Ida and pingala nadis tasks in the three main parts of the nervous system.

A sensory-motor nervous system is where all electrical activity in the body moves within two paths. Into the brain (afferent), ida, and through the brain (efferent), pingala.

The Chakranas
Colour Nr. of Petals Yantra
Action Element & Bija mantra

Sahasrara chakra – I understand
Dark red. 1000 petals. Aum. Shiva

Ajna chakra
White, 2 Petals
Pyramid

Third Eye
I see
Moon Aum

Vishuddhi chakra
Purple 16 petals
Cirkel with Space

I talk
Space Element
mantra Ham

Anahata chakra.
Blue, 12 petals
Blue Davidstar

I love
Air element
mantra Yam

Manipura chakra
Yellow, 10 petals
Red triangel

I do
Fire element
mantra Ram

Swadhisthana c.
Orange, 10 petals
Half moon

I feel
Water element
mantra Vam

Mooladhara chakra – I am
Red 4 petals. Bija mantra Lam
Earth element, Yellow square

The autonomic nervous system is divided into the outward, stress management, energy utilization, Pingala dominant, sympathetic nervous system, and inward, relaxed, energy saving, ida dominant parasympathetic nervous system. The central nervous system consists of the brain and spine, which controls the two preceding parts of the nervous system.

The yogic techniques are based on the knowledge of our nadis and chakras. The physical experience of these is that you can also experience it physically through the different parts of the nervous system. The nervous system's influence on our physical body describes the importance of balancing and harmonizing the flow between ida, pingala, and sushumna nadi.

THE IMPORTANCE OF PREPARATION, EXERCISE, AND NOT TAKING WATER OVER YOUR HEAD

As a beginner in yoga full of desire and inspiration, it is easy to get water over your head. Yoga is a process in which the body and mind are prepared for more advanced techniques. It's like running. If you have run several marathons, you may need longer stretches to feel the training gives something. You, as a new runner, benefit from running three kilometers. This is precisely how yoga works.

When you have practiced Hatha yoga for a few years, feel comfortable in the positions with all the locks and postures, and master the breathing exercises, you can move on with the most advanced tantric techniques. Then, they will not feel too complicated, and you will have a consciousness that allows you to enjoy the effects of your practice without it becoming too much. If something feels too difficult, go back one step instead. Everything comes to you when you are ready. Hurry slowly.

"YOU EXPERIENCE ALL THE POWER
IN THE COSMOS AND ON EARTH,
IN YOURSELF AND AROUND.
EVERYTHING YOU WANT IS POSSIBLE
BECAUSE ALL POWER IS YOURS!"

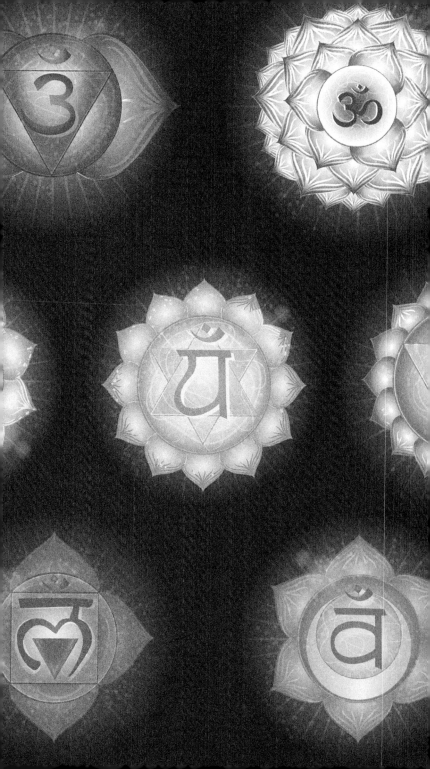

CHAKRANA
INDEX

AJNA CHAKRA

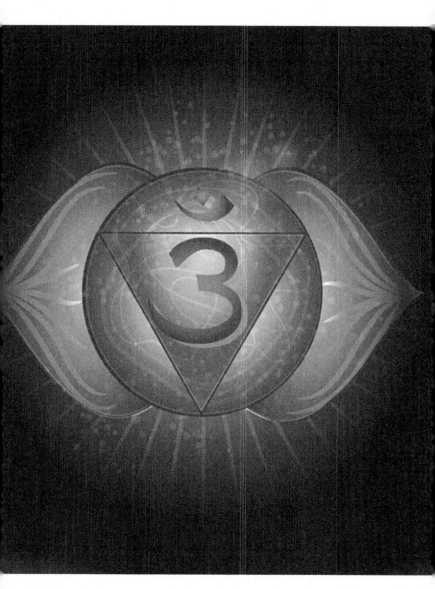

AJNA CHAKRA

TANMATRA *(a sensory experience):* Sense.

JNANENDRIYA *(sense organ):* Sense.

KARMENDRIYA *(body of action):* Sense.

TATTWA *(element):* Sense.

BIJA MANTRA *Om.*

TATTWA SYMBOL *Picture of the mantra Om.*

YOGA TYPE *Jnana, Raja and Mantra yoga (Sattvic).*

LOTUS (PADMA) *White, silver, or smoky with two petals.*

AJNA CHAKRA *(third eye) is associated with the mind, reason, intelligence, and intuition. It is also the center through which two people, through the intellect – on a deeper level, are in contact with each other—for example, the touch between guru (teacher/master) and student / disciple.*

Direct concentration on the Ajna chakra is challenging. Therefore, one focuses on tantra and yoga in the middle of the eyebrow center (the kshetram of the Ajna chakra). This point is called bhrumadhya (bhru- refers to eyebrows, and madhya refers to the center) and lies between the eyebrows where Indian ladies put a red dot, and Pandits and Brahmins put a mark. Various techniques can touch this eyebrow center.

Ajna and Mooladhara chakras are closely related, and awakening in one of these helps to awaken the others. Ideally, Ajna should be awakened to some extent before Mooladhara to prepare the mind for all the hidden memories and impressions that come to the surface as we practice chakra awakening. But the awakening in Mooladhara will also help to awaken Ajna further. The best way to bring about the awakening of Ajna is moola bandha and Ashwini mudra, which are specific to Mooladhara.

The Ajna chakra and the pineal gland are the same, just like the pituitary gland is the physical aspect of Sahasrara. The pituitary gland and the pineal gland are intimately connected, as are the Ajna and Sahasrara. Ajna is the gateway to the Sahasrara chakra. If Ajna is awakened and works, then all experiences in Sahasrara happen as well.

The pineal gland acts as a lock for the pituitary gland. As long as the pineal gland is healthy, the pituitary gland works on a deeper, spiritual level. But for most of us, the pineal gland stops developing when we turn eight, nine, or ten years old, and this is when the pituitary gland begins to function and secrete various hormones that stimulate our sexual consciousness, sensuality, and worldly person. At this time, we started to lose touch with our spiritual heritage. However, through various yogic techniques, such as trataka and Shambhavi mudra, it is possible to restore or maintain the health of the pineal gland. The pineal gland and Ajna chakra have a special significance in esoteric yoga and tantra. It is where siddhis (occult / magical) abilities are manifested.

The "third eye" is a mysterious and esoteric concept referring to Ajna chakra in various spiritual traditions from the East and West. It is also said to be a door that leads into inner worlds and stages of higher consciousness. In tantra and yoga, the "third eye" can symbolize enlightenment or the development of mental images with deeply spiritual or psychological meanings. The "third eye" is often associated with siddhis, such as revelations, prophecy (including the ability to observe chakras and auras), divination, and out-of-body experiences. A person considered to have developed an ability to use his "third eye" is called a Siddha in yoga and is referred to as someone who has acquired siddhis.

HANDS-ON YOGA TECHNIQUES FOR AJNA CHAKRA ACTI-VATING AND PURIFICATION

To practice regularly for a month.

Suppose you have difficulty connecting with the chakra's pulsation and can identify with impaired intuition. In that case, there are powerful yogic techniques to cleanse, balance, and activate the chakra. It would be best if you did them regularly for the specified time, and it is recommended that you also follow a healthy, balancing yoga routine to strengthen the effect. Find a form of yoga that you like, and that is at the appropriate level. Avoid caffeine, white sugar, red meat, and stress and energy stealers as much as possible. Also, reduce your internet /mobile usage and give yourself the chance for natural healing. Good luck!

Practice 15-30 minutes.

Shambhavi mudra with Om chanting.
Chakra and kshetram localization / activation and purification through Shambhavi mudra with Om chanting (open eyes – fast Om, then close your eyes and inhale slowly – O … in through bhrumadhya (eyebrow center) … out with M …) Experience the pulsation from the chakra and visualize the color. You can also visualize the yantra.

Anuloma viloma pranayama.
Anuloma viloma pranayama alt. prana shuddhi. Inhale through the left nostril, exhale through the right nostril and count to 1. Inhale through the right nostril and out through the left and count to 1. Inhale through the left nostril and count to 2; exhale through the right and count to 2. Etc. On 5, 10, and 15, etc., you inhale through both and out through both nostrils. If you lose the count, you start again from 1.

Trataka.

Trataka. Light a candle and sit in a meditation position with a straight back. Squint at the light, do not fully close your eyes. Look at the embers in the flame for 30 seconds, then close your eyes and look at the after-image of the flame behind your closed eyes ...

"THE PINEAL GLAND ...
AND THE DMT MOLECULE - THE THIRD EYE ...
THERE MAY BE A WAY FOR THE BRAIN TO TAKE US TO
A HIGHER PLANE OF EXISTENCE, WHERE WE CAN
UNDERSTAND THE WORLD AND OUR RELATIONSHIPS
TO THINGS AND PEOPLE ON A DEEPER LEVEL AND
WHERE WE CAN ULTIMATELY CREATE A DEEPER
MEANING FOR OURSELVES AND OUR WORLD.
THERE IS A SPIRITUAL PART OF THE BRAIN - IT IS A
PART THAT WE CAN ALL HAVE ACCESS TO AND IS
SOMETHING WE ALL CAN ACCOMPLISH."

(ANDREW NEWBERG - BRAIN RESEARCHER)

MOOLADHARA CHAKRA

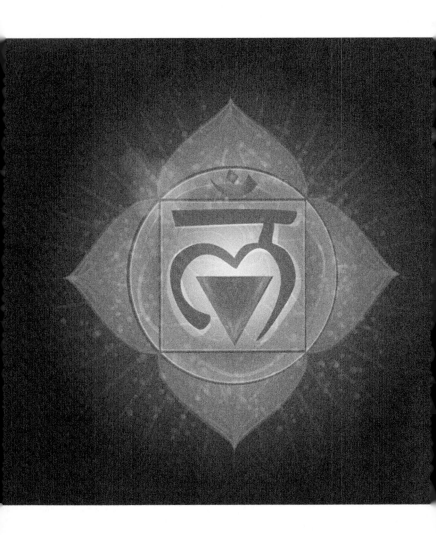

MOOLADHARA CHAKRA

TANMATRA *(a sensory experience): Smell.*

JNANENDRIYA *(sense organ): Nose.*

KARMENDRIYA *(organ of action): Anus.*

TATTWA *(element): Prithvi (earth).*

BIJA MANTRA *Lam.*

TATTWA SYMBOL *Yellow square.*

ANIMALS *Elephant.*

YOGA TYPE *Tantra and Hatha yoga (counteracts tamas / inertia).*

LOTUS (PADMA) *Red lotus with four petals.*

MOOLADHARA CHAKRA

Moola means root – a triangular space in the middle of the body at a point between the genitals and anus for men and at the cervix for women. Mooladhara chakra is associated with personal security in both thought and action. At this level, the individual focuses mainly on obtaining food and shelter and securing his reproduction. To create personal security, she surrounds herself with material things, money, family, and friends.

In the middle of Mooladhara, one usually imagines a black swayam-

bhu linga (a symbol of male power, Shiva). Around this, the serpent
Kundalini (Shakti, the mother of all prana in the human body) winds
three and a half turns – dozing in anticipation of its awakening, as it
ascends through sushumna nadi to unite with Shiva in Sahasrara Pad-
ma in the moment of enlightenment. This event can only happen when
the individual's spiritual development is mature.

MOOLADHARA'S IMPACT ON OUR DIFFERENT BODIES

IN ANNAMAYA KOSHA *(physical body).*
Reproductive organs, perineum, uterine tube.

IN PRANAMAYA KOSHA *(energy body).*
Apana vayu.

IN MANOMAYA KOSHA *(body of thought).*
Security, ownership, safety, survival.

MOOLADHARA IN DIFFERENT STAGES OF GUNAS
Creation and its energy consist of three gunas, fundamental properties
or tendencies: sattva, rajas, and tamas. These three gunas act and react
incessantly with each other. The world of phenomena is composed of
different combinations of these three gunas. Tamas stands for inertia,
rajas for movement, and sattva for balance. When Mooladhara is ba-
lanced and sattvic, we are safe and secure in ourselves and the world.
When Mooladhara is out of balance and is tamasic, we experience
boundless fear. We are in a deep psychosis. As the balance becomes
more rajasic, our condition changes, as shown below. The yogi believes
he can alleviate and dissolve negative states by identifying one's form
with the right degree of imbalance / balance in the various chakras.

TAMAS *Horror.*

TAMAS / RAJAS *Anxiety, worries.*

RAJAS / TAMAS *Greed, self-confidence.*
RAJAS *Collector.*

RAJAS / SATTVA *Generosity.*

SATTVA / RAJAS *Property for good cause.*

SATTVA *Safe in the physical world.*

ENLIGHTENED *Unity with the absolute.*

HANDS-ON YOGA TECHNIQUES FOR MOOLADHARA CHAKRA ACTIVATING AND PURIFICATION

To practice regularly for a month.

Suppose you have difficulty connecting with the chakra's pulsation and can identify with the imbalances described. In that case, there are powerful yogic techniques to cleanse, balance, and activate the chakra. It would be best if you did them regularly for the specified time, and it is recommended that you also follow a healthy, balancing yoga routine to strengthen the effect. Find a form of yoga that you like, and that is at the appropriate level. Avoid caffeine, white sugar, red meat, and stress and energy stealers as much as possible. Also, reduce your internet / mobile usage and give yourself the chance for natural healing.

Practice 15-30 minutes.

Moola bandha with bija mantra Lam.

Chakra and kshetram localization / activation and purification by Moola bandha, contraction of the abdomen, first slowly; breathe in – hold the breath … feel the pulsation a few centimeters up from the diaphragm inside the body and pronounce the mantra Lam in time with the pulse beat and then release the lock … then quickly and with Lam in step with breathing. Then, sit for about five minutes with a powerful Moola bandha and feel the pulsation of the chakra and chant Lam. You can also visualize the color and yantra.

Nasikagra drishti – focus on the tip of the nose.

Nasikagra drishti – focus on the nose tip without closing your eyes. If your eyes get tired during this exercise, you can close them briefly and then return to the exercise.

SWADHISTHANA

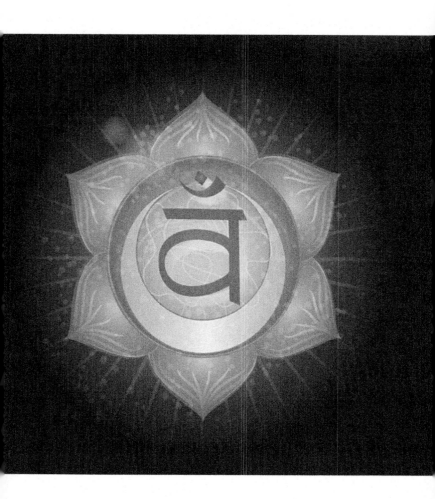

SWADHISTHANA CHAKRA

TANMATRA *(a sensory experience): Taste.*

JNANENDRIYA *(sense organ): Tongue.*

KARMENDRIYA *(organ of action): Genitals.*

TATTWA *(element): Apas (water).*

BIJA MANTRA *Vam.*

TATTWA SYMBOL *White crescent.*

ANIMALS *Crocodile.*

YOGA TYPE *Tantra and Hatha yoga (counteracts tamas / inertia).*

LOTUS (PADMA) *Orange lotus with six petals.*

SWADHISTHANA CHAKRA *(pleasure, lust)*
The chakra sits at the base of the spine just inside the lower tailbone and at the height of the genitals. Chakra is associated with sensory experiences. One strives to achieve sensory enjoyment through, e.g., food, drinks, sex, etc. You value everything in terms of the enjoyment you can thereby achieve. The difference from the Mooladhara chakra is that here, we strive for the pleasure of the mind rather than for satisfying basic needs.

It is said that most people in the world primarily act and are motivated at this level. Swadhisthana chakra is also usually associated with the unconscious. It is noted that coexistence – traces or patterns created in the unconscious of our experiences and actions we perform – have their place in this chakra. Samskaras eventually form the basis of the individual's karma. Most of these cohabitants are displaced from consciousness or can even be repressed. Therefore, the Swadhisthana chakra is often associated with desires, urges, and fears over which we have no control.

THE IMPACT OF SWADHISTHANA ON OUR DIFFERENT BODIES

ANNAMAYA KOSHA *(physical body): Genitals, urination.*

PRANAMAYA KOSHA *(energy body): Apana vayu.*

MANOMAYA KOSHA *(body of thought): Satisfaction, pleasure, sex (from happiness to addiction).*

SWADHISTHANA IN DIFFERENT STAGES OF GUNAS

TAMAS *Depression.*

TAMAS / RAJAS *Bitterness, the feeling of being rejected.*

RAJAS / TAMAS *Desire, sexual exploitation.*

RAJAS *Seeking pleasure, sexual conquests.*

RAJAS / SATTVA *Humor, caring sexuality with love.*

SATTVA / RAJAS *Happily satisfied.*

SATTVA *Bubbly happy.*

ENLIGHTENED *Ananda, happiness "bliss."*

HANDS-ON YOGA TECHNIQUES FOR SWADHISTHANA CHAKRA ACTIVATING AND PURIFICATION

To practice regularly for a month.

Suppose you have difficulty connecting with the chakra's pulsation and can identify with the imbalances described. In that case, there are powerful yogic techniques to cleanse, balance, and activate the chakra. It would be best if you did them regularly for the specified time, and it is recommended that you also follow a healthy, balancing yoga routine to strengthen the effect. Find a form of yoga that you like, and that is at the appropriate level. Avoid caffeine, white sugar, red meat, and stress and energy stealers as much as possible. Also, reduce your internet / mobile usage and give yourself the chance for natural healing.

Practice 15-30 minutes.

Ashwini mudra with bija mantra Vam.

Chakra and kshetram localization, activation, and purification. For the chakra: Ashwini mudra – first slowly. Inhale, contract the rectum, and hold your breath ... feel the pulsation with Vam in the chakra a few centimeters up from the end of the tailbone ... then quickly and with Vam in time with breathing.

Vajroli (or sahajoli) mudra with bija mantra Vam.

For kshetram: Vajroli (or sahajoli) mudra – first slowly. Inhale and contract the genitals and hold your breath ... feel the pulsation with Vam at the kshetram for the chakra at the genitals ... then quickly and with Vam in time with breathing.

MANIPURA CHAKRA

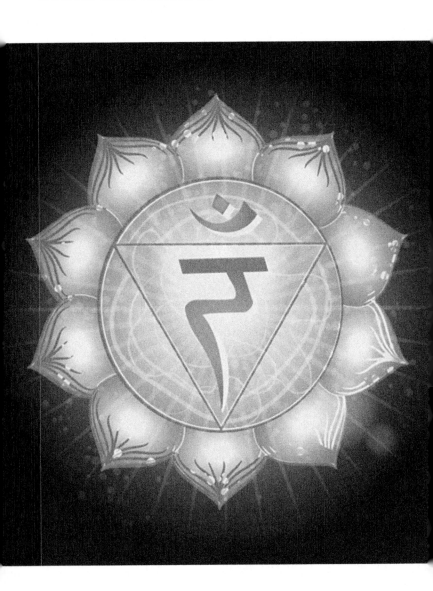

MANIPURA CHAKRA

TANMATRA *(a sensory experience): Vision.*

JNANENDRIYA *(sensory organs): Eyes.*

KARMENDRIYA *(organ of action): Feet.*

TATTWA *(element): Agni (fire).*

BIJA MANTRA *Ram.*

TATTWA SYMBOL *Red inverted triangle.*

ANIMALS *Aries.*

YOGA TYPE *Karma yoga (counteracts rajas / mobility).*

LOTUS (PADMA) *Yellow lotus with ten petals.*

MANIPURA *(seat of the jewel).*
The chakra is located in the spine at the level of the navel. It is associated with will, worldly pursuit, ambition, and career. Man grows as a social and self-conscious being from the energy of manipulation. She cultivates material desires, such as owning and mastering power, prestige, and usefulness. But also selflessness, social balance, and prosperity.

Manipura's energy is outward and active, a vital energy that provides the power to act and change oneself and one's surroundings. Someti-

mes, this happens with a selfish attitude where other people are seen as a means to achieve their ambition, but here, the first expressions of a growing self-awareness begin to take shape in man. The ego is still dominant, but the first traces of a genuine, spiritual pursuit are manifested at this level. One begins to question one's existence and one's motives seriously.

THE IMPACT OF MANIPURA ON OUR DIFFERENT BODIES

ANNAMAYA KOSHA *(physical body): Solar Plexus, digestion.*

PRANAMAYA KOSHA *(energy body): Samana vayu.*

MANOMAYA KOSHA *(body of thought): Power, action, self-confidence and striving.*

MANIPURA IN DIFFERENT STAGES OF GUNAS

TAMAS *Inability to act.*

TAMAS / RAJAS *Guilt over non-actions, low self-esteem.*

RAJAS / TAMAS *Frustration over one's inability.*

RAJAS *Active, brave.*

RAJAS / SATTVA *Anxious, ready to act.*

SATTVA / RAJAS *Karma yoga at an intermediate level.*

SATTVA *Things happen as if by miracle.*

ENLIGHTENED: *Omnipotent.*

HANDS-ON YOGA TECHNIQUES FOR MANIPURA CHAKRA ACTIVATING AND PURIFICATION

To practice regularly for a month.

Suppose you have difficulty connecting with the chakra's pulsation and can identify with the imbalances described. In that case, there are powerful yogic techniques to cleanse, balance, and activate the chakra. It would be best if you did them regularly for the specified time, and it is recommended that you also follow a healthy, balancing yoga routine to strengthen the effect. Find a form of yoga that you like, and that is at the appropriate level. Avoid caffeine, white sugar, red meat, and stress and energy stealers as much as possible. Also, reduce your internet / mobile usage and give yourself the chance for natural healing.

Uddiyana bandha with bija mantra Ram.
Chakra and kshetram localization / activation and purification through uddiyana bandha / belly lock with Ram chanting. Inhale, hold your breath as you inhale using the diaphragm, and practice the stomach lock / uddiyana bandha. Experience the pulsation from the chakra and visualize the color while you say Ram quietly to yourself. You can also visualize the yantra.

Bhastrika and kapalbhati with uddiyana bandha.
Inhale and expand your stomach, exhale and contract – bhastrika; practice this for about 30 rounds, then hold your breath out, lean forward on straight arms with your hands on your knees, and practice stomach locks. The same technique applies to kapalbhati, but now you put all the focus on the exhalation and let the inhalation take care of itself.

Union with prana and apana vayu.

Sit in a meditation position and experience how prana vayu moves down to the navel and unites with apana vayu, which moves up from the anus to the navel on inhalation. Exhale, and the energy currents turn and move up and down the body. Continue for about 5 minutes.

ANAHATA CHAKRA

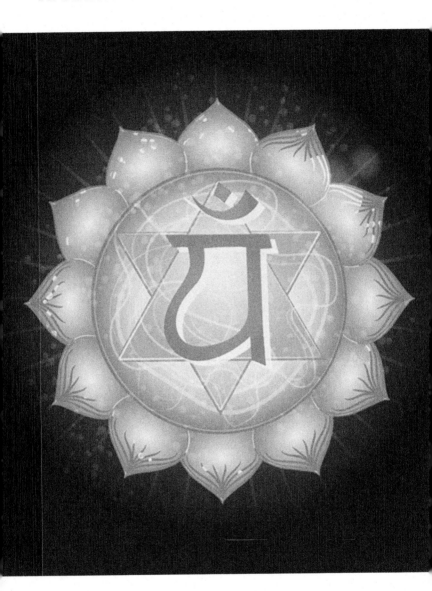

ANAHATA CHAKRA

TANMATRA *(a sensory experience): Feeling.*

JNANENDRIYA *(sense organ): Skin.*

KARMENDRIYA *(body of action): Hands.*

TATTWA *(element): Vayu (air).*

BIJA MANTRA *Yam.*

TATTWA SYMBOL *Blue hexagram.*

ANIMALS *Black antelope.*

YOGA TYPE *Bhakti and Karma yoga (counteracts rajas / mobility).*

LOTUS (PADMA) *Blue or green lotus with twelve petals.*

ANAHATA *(unspoken "sound," the origin of all mantras). Anahata sits in the spine at the height of the heart. Its energy is associated with love, hate, joy, sorrow, and the beauty experience. Chakra is strongly related to our relationships with others around us.*

At this level, the individual often begins to love everything and everyone unconditionally. You learn to ignore the faults and shortcomings of others and take them for what they are. Anahata also stands for aesthetic discernment and artistic creation. The energy is expressed here in

the form of creativity, regardless of which area you are active in. At this
level, man leaves the material world to cultivate higher values.

THE INFLUENCE OF ANAHATA IN OUR DIFFERENT BODIES

ANNAMAYA KOSHA *(physical body): Heart, lungs.*

PRANAMAYA KOSHA *(energy body): Vyana vayu.*

MANOMAYA KOSHA *(body of thought): Love, compassion, acceptance and tolerance.*

ANAHATA IN DIFFERENT STAGES OF GUNAS

TAMAS *Apathy.*

TAMAS / RAJAS *Fraud, treason.*

RAJAS / TAMAS *Avoid intimacy.*

RAJAS *Love under certain conditions.*

RAJAS / SATTVA *Care about others.*

SATTVA / RAJAS *Love and compassion.*

SATTVA *Is love.*

ENLIGHTENED *Cosmic love.*

HANDS-ON YOGA TECHNIQUES FOR ANAHATA CHAKRA ACTIVATING AND PURIFICATION

To practice regularly for a month.

Suppose you have difficulty connecting with the chakra's pulsation and can identify with the imbalances described. In that case, there are powerful yogic techniques to cleanse, balance, and activate the chakra. It would be best if you did them regularly for the specified time, and it is recommended that you also follow a healthy, balancing yoga routine to strengthen the effect. Find a form of yoga that you like, and that is at the appropriate level. Avoid caffeine, white sugar, red meat, and stress and energy stealers as much as possible. Also, reduce your internet / mobile usage and give yourself the chance for natural healing.

Yam chanting.

Chakra and kshetram localization / activation & purification with Yam chanting. Press one finger against the heart and one finger at the corresponding point at the spine. Inhale and hold your breath as you experience the pulsation from the chakra and visualize the color while saying Yam silently to yourself. You can also visualize the yantra. Exhale and then continue in the same way for 5-10 minutes.

Anahata chakra bhedan.

Anahata chakra bhedan i matsyasana. Practice matsyasana (the fish), inhale through the heart, and pierce the spine and chakras. Feel how the astral body expands like a hot air balloon, and you experience the chakra attributes. You feel light – lighter than air; you float high up in the clouds, experience the blue sky, and experience boundless love and happiness throughout your body, eternal joy in every little cell. When you exhale – you exhale through the spine and heart, and the body contracts slightly. Continue for 2-5 minutes.

VISHUDDHI CHAKRA

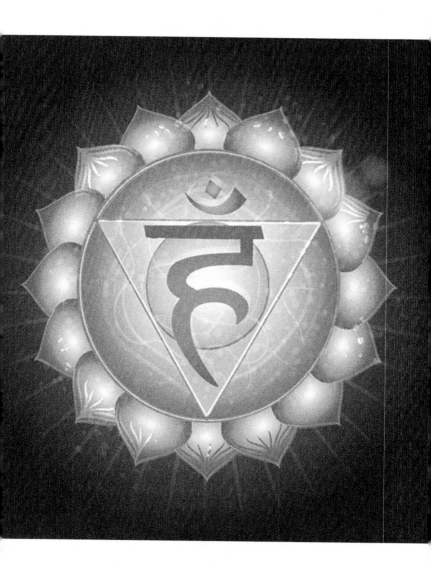

VISHUDDHI CHAKRA

TANMATRA *(a sensory experience): Sound.*

JNANENDRIYA *(sensory organs): Ears.*

KARMENDRIYA *(body of action): Body of speech.*

TATTWA *(element): Akasha (space).*

BIJA MANTRA *Ham.*

TATTWA SYMBOL *White and black circle.*

ANIMALS *White elephant.*

YOGA TYPE *Jnana, Raja and Mantra yoga (sattvic).*

LOTUS (PADMA) *Violet lotus with sixteen petals.*

VISHUDDHI *(purity).*
The chakra sits in the neck behind the larynx. It is associated with an attitude of independence (vairagya), where both pleasant and unpleasant aspects of human life are seen and accepted as rewarding experiences. The world appears as a place full of harmony and perfection. Everything you experience, good or bad, is seen as part of a whole that helps remove personal problems, locks, and limitations and raise consciousness. This attitude leads to discernment (viveka).

Vishuddhi is also associated with expression, communication in general, and the spoken word in particular.

THE IMPACT OF VISHUDDHI ON OUR DIFFERENT BODIES

ANNAMAYA KOSHA *(physical body): The thyroid gland, parathyroid gland, trachea and esophagus.*

PRANAMAYA KOSHA *(energy body): Udana vayu.*

MANOMAYA KOSHA *(body of thought): Communication.*

VISHUDDHI IN DIFFERENT STAGES OF GUNAS

TAMAS *Isolated.*

TAMAS / RAJAS *Limited contact / communication.*

RAJAS / TAMAS *Complaining/whining.*

RAJAS *Pretty good communicator.*

RAJAS / SATTVA *Eloquent.*

SATTVA / RAJAS *Persuader, non-violent communication.*

SATTVA *True communication.*

ENLIGHTENED *Cosmic communication.*

HANDS-ON YOGA TECHNIQUES FOR VISHUDDHI CHAKRA ACTIVATING AND PURIFICATION

To practice regularly for a month.

Suppose you have difficulty connecting with the chakra's pulsation and can identify with the imbalances described. In that case, there are powerful yogic techniques to cleanse, balance, and activate the chakra. It would be best if you did them regularly for the specified time, and it is recommended that you also follow a healthy, balancing yoga routine to strengthen the effect. Find a form of yoga that you like, and that is at the appropriate level. Avoid caffeine, white sugar, red meat, and stress and energy stealers as much as possible. Also, reduce your internet / mobile usage and give yourself the chance for natural healing.

Chakra and kshetram localization/activation and purification with Ham chanting.

Press one finger against the neck and one finger at the corresponding point on the other side of the neck. Inhale and hold your breath as you experience the pulsation from the chakra and visualize the color while saying Ham silently to yourself. You can also visualize the yantra. Exhale and then continue in the same way for 5-10 minutes.

BINDU VISARGA

Bindu visarga is located on top of the back of the head. Many claim that one can not find Bindu in the physical body but can only be experienced via nada, i.e., via its vibration or sound. It is not a chakra in the ordinary sense.

Through techniques like moorcha pranayama and vajroli / sahajoli mudra, we can develop the experience of nada. Through methods like bhramari pranayama and shanmukhi mudra, we can follow nada to its source – Bindu.

There is a close relationship between the Swadhisthana chakra and the Bindu because Bindu is the point where the vibration and sound of the individual creation are first manifested, and Swadhisthana is the center of composition in the form of sexual reproduction. Swadhisthana expresses our physical desire for union with the cosmic consciousness. Sperm and menstruation are physical expressions of the drops of Amrit – the nectar drops of creation or secretions that drip from the Bindu and are burned in the Manipura chakra via the Vishuddhi chakra. The drops control the creation process and the body's aging.

It is commonly believed that Bindu Visarga has no kshetram – contact point.

HANDS-ON YOGA TECHNIQUES FOR BINDU VISARGA ACTIVATING AND PURIFICATION

To practice regularly for a month.

Suppose you have difficulty connecting with the chakra's pulsation and sound. In that case, there are powerful yogic techniques to cleanse, balance, and activate the chakra. It would be best if you did them regularly for the specified time, and it is recommended that you also follow a healthy, balancing yoga routine to strengthen the effect. Find a form of yoga that you like, and that is at the appropriate level. Avoid caffeine, white sugar, red meat, and stress and energy stealers as much as possible. Also, reduce your internet / mobile usage and give yourself the chance for natural healing.

Moorcha pranayama.

Sit in a meditation position. Practice kechari mudra. Inhale – slowly and deeply, through both nostrils with ujjayi pranayama while tilting your head back and performing shambhavi mudra. Experience the Bindu. Keep your arms straight by pressing your hands against your knees. Then, bend your arms while slowly exhaling with ujjayi, pointing your head forward, and closing your eyes. Then relax completely and experience a sensation of lightness and calm in the body—about ten rounds or more.

Vajroli / sahajoli mudra with concentration on Bindu.

Sit in a meditation position. Squeeze the urethra without activating the ashwini mudra or moola bandha. Pinch for 10 seconds, and relax for 10 seconds. Continue like this for about 5 minutes. Every time you pinch, you experience Swadhisthana chakra at the tailbone and say – Swadhisthana 3 times. Then go via sushumna up to Bindu and

say – Bindu, 3 times. Then, return to Swadhisthana and relax. Up to
25 rounds. NOTE. In this context, this exercise should be practiced
directly after the moorcha pranayama as these activate and locate the
Bindu visarga together.

The experience of the inner sound.

Practice the bumblebee first – bhramari pranayama, for a while. 5-10
minutes. Put your index fingers in your ears, close your eyes, and hum
quietly. Then, sit in the same sitting position with your index fingers
in your ears and be completely silent. Listen for the first best sound
in your head. Then, isolate this sound. You use this sound to increase
your consciousness. Just experience this sound – nothing else. After a
while, you can hear an even more subtle sound in the background –
then you concentrate on this sound and gradually use the same techni-
que to penetrate more deeply into the subtle vibrations of the head—10
minutes or more.

Shanmukhi mudra.

Siddhasana / siddha yoni asana. Sit on a pillow that touches the
Mooladhara chakra. Relax. Then, use your fingers to close your ears
(thumb), eyes (index finger), nose (middle finger), and mouth (ring &
little fingers). Then release the pressure against the nostrils – inhale,
close again with your fingers, and hold your breath. Listen to sounds
from the Bindu, the middle of the head, or the ears. Then, go from the
rough sounds to the fine ones. Keep going for a short time at a sound.
5-10 minutes. Shanmukhi mudra means – to close the 7 openings (to
the outer world and start listening to the inner – mind).

SAHASRARA CHAKRA

The chakra is located just above the head and is purple / red. It has a thousand petals and represents pure consciousness. When Kundalini Shakti reaches the Sahasrara chakra, we become enlightened, and according to yoga, we enter nirvikalpa samadhi.

The function of the Sahasrara is to provide us with other levels of consciousness, which may make us realize that "we are one" and that "everything is one." Through the crown chakra, we experience union with God and the supernatural. The Crown chakra is what is called "pure consciousness."

When one reaches a higher level of consciousness in this chakra, all thinking is released. Here lay the answers to all our questions, the absolute truth that we all dream of getting answers to, and where we find total freedom – We become enlightened.

HANDS-ON YOGA TECHNIQUES FOR SAHASRARA ACTIVATING AND PURIFICATION

To practice regularly for a month.

Suppose you have difficulty connecting with the chakra's pulsation and experiences of heightened awareness. In that case, there are powerful yogic techniques to cleanse, balance, and activate the chakra. It would be best if you did them regularly for the specified time, and it is recommended that you also follow a healthy, balancing yoga routine to strengthen the effect. Find a form of yoga that you like, and that is at the appropriate level. Avoid caffeine, white sugar, red meat, and stress and energy stealers as much as possible. Also, reduce your internet / mobile usage and give yourself the chance for natural healing.

Chakra and kshetram localization / activation and purification with Aum chanting.

Press one finger against the top of the head. Inhale and hold your breath as you experience the pulsation from the chakra and visualize the color while saying Aum silently to yourself. Exhale and then continue in the same way for 5-10 minutes.

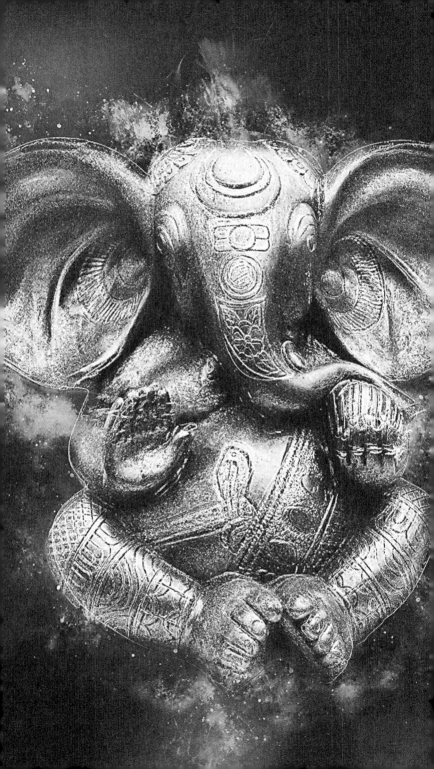

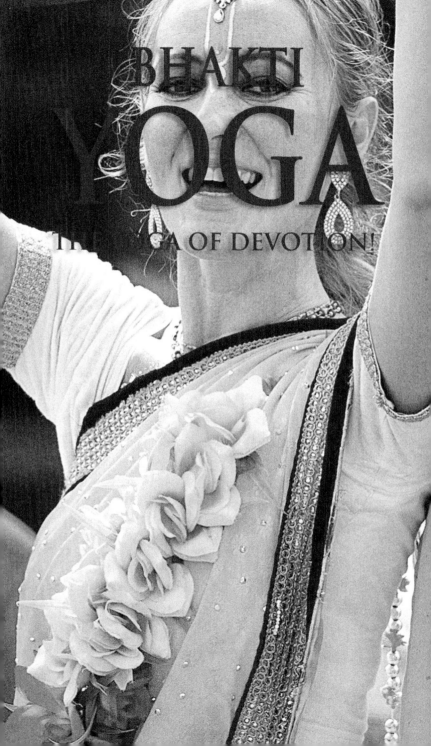

BHAKTI
YOGA

THE YOGA OF DEVOTION!

KARMA, BHAKTI
& JNANA YOGA

HINDUISM

Hinduism differs from other religions in that it can be described as a collective name for a host of religious denominations that lack a common core. Most Hindus see Hinduism as a set of ritual acts, something practiced. But Hinduism is also a tradition that carries an extensive collection of knowledge – it is the religion with the most significant number of sacred texts.

In Hinduism, humans are perceived as thinking, biological, and social beings characterized by people's different interests and aptitudes for things. They worship different gods, read other texts, follow different teaching systems and gurus, and visit various temples. This view is the basis for the hierarchical method applied in Hinduism and the tolerance for each other's differences and diversity.

Diversity expresses the process of change and development that Prakriti undergoes. On the other hand, Purusha is what all individuals have in common – the unchanging self, the atman, as the Samkhya philosophy describes.

Samkhya and yoga both belong to the philosophical system of Hinduism. The purpose of the systems is to guide man towards moksha, or freedom from the cycle of rebirth. Moksha is considered the fourth and final goal in a person's life.

The six philosophical systems are arranged in doctrinal pairs as follows:

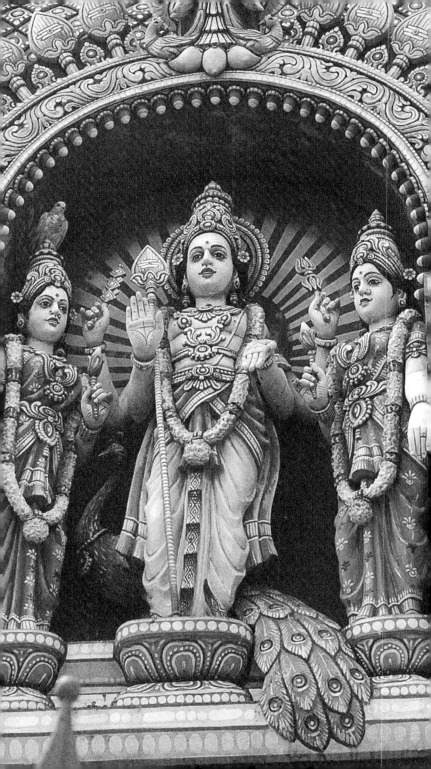

Nyaya – logic.
Vaisheshika – atomic.

Samkhya – cosmic principle.
Yoga – Yoga.

Purva-Mimamsa (Vedanta) – ritual.
Uttara-Mimamsa (Vedanta) – theological.

The belief within these systems of a person's ability to be liberated differs from the bhakti-oriented theistic Vedan schools, whose adherents believe that a person depends on God's grace to be free from the cycle of rebirth.

Samkhya and yoga are described together in many of the Hindu texts, indicating an early connection to each other.

The Katha, Svetasvatara, and Maitri Upanishads describe yogic exercises and Samkhya together. In the Katha Upanishad, yoga is used as a means of meditation. Yoga and Samkhya are also mentioned in close connection in the Mahabharata. Here, the goal of yoga is described as the realization of the atman (the self) and Brahman (matter).

The Bhagavad Gita, part of the Mahabharata, describes yoga in three ways – Jnana, Karma, and Bhakti yoga. Krishna is seen here as the master of yoga.

The Yoga Sutras of Patanjali, an essential text in Hinduism and the most important work of classical yoga, has become and serve as a basic description. Here, too, Samkhya plays a central role. Even yoga traditions that do not share the same view of the ultimate reality have embraced the Yoga Sutras, which describe them logically and coherently. In the Yoga Sutras, yoga is defined as the cessation of the mind's activities, which we today call meditation.

DHARMA

A central concept in Hinduism is dharma, likened to duty, law, rightness, and firmness. Many Hindus today call their religion Sanatana dharma (the eternal dharma). Dharma is the eternal order, and in the oldest scriptures, it refers to the various rituals and duties performed to maintain social and cosmic order.

Dharma is based on the notion that humans maintain the universe through actions. Various rituals, civil and criminal law, stages of life, pilgrimages, sacrifices, etc, cover these actions. Dharma is used to structure society and the life of the individual. It plays a significant role in the caste systems applied in Hindu culture.

Following one's dharma should lead to a better rebirth and be a path to ultimate salvation.

TRADITIONS

The core tradition of Hinduism is Brahmanical, the most dominant and widespread practice in India. Men in the tradition are authoritarian. The Vedic texts play a central role and are seen as revelations. The tradition includes the priesthood, a sacred language (Sanskrit), and the perception of a holy social order. Rituals are performed in temples and ceremonies in the home. Hindu deities such as Shiva, Vishnu, Rama, Krishna, Durga, Kali, and Ganesha are worshipped. Pilgrimages, festivals, rules about food, and cleanliness are also important.

The other primary focus is organizations, where the focus is usually on moksha (salvation). These typically have a founder, and some are more ritually oriented (Sri Vishnuism and Sri Vidya), while others function as organizations for ascetics (Vishnuite: Ramanandi and Nada; or Shivaite: Natha and Aghori). They are often bearers of different yoga traditions, and men from the Brahmin class are often seen as leaders of these groups.

The guru movements also belong to this tradition; these often have to compete for followers. Many have also succeeded in communicating their teachings internationally, such as Maharishi Mahesh Yogi (Transcendental Meditation) and A.C. Bhaktivedanta Swami Prabhupada (International Society for Krishna Consciousness).

A third focus is the village and tribe-based traditions of India. Priests in this tradition are not from the Brahmin class, and gods with a local connection are worshipped. The Brahmin core tradition sees these practices as unclean, which has led to a tense relationship.

VISHNUISM, SHIVAISM AND SHAKTISM

Sacrifice rituals were a central part of the Brahmanic tradition but became less important as the ascetic ideology emerged. Knowledge and renunciation became more critical than being freed from the cycle of rebirth. Many influential gods in the Vedic sacrificial tradition fell away, while Shiva and Vishnu remained important. Groups sprang up where one of these gods was worshipped, laying the foundation for Hinduism. The ritual worship of gods (puja) that then arose competed with the sacrificial culture (yajna).

Seventy percent of Hindus worship Vishnu or one of his avatars, such

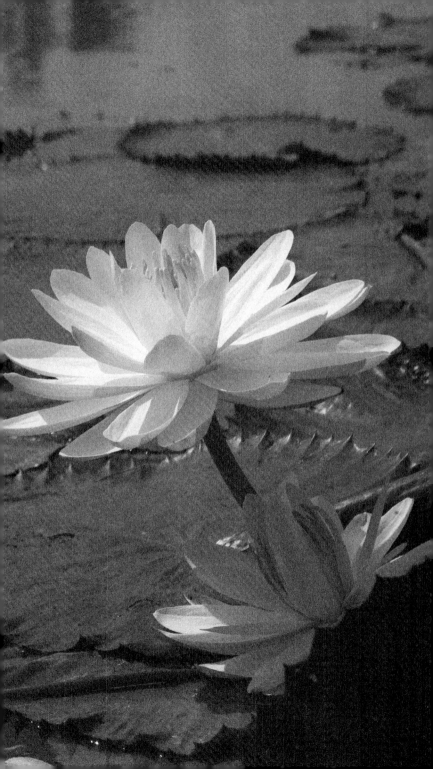

as Rama or Krishna. Vishnu's task is to sustain the world. In the form of Krishna, he evokes feelings of love and care. In the form of Rama, he symbolizes the world order, dharma, and the dutiful man. Worship and devotion to a personal god is what characterizes Vishnuism. Still, there are also organizations for ascetics, and some groups have taken up some tantrism and instead worshipped a goddess such as Lakshmi.

Twenty-eight percent of Hindus worship Shiva, his family members, his wife Parvati, and their sons Ganesha and Skanda. Shiva is a great yogi and a friendly god, but he also has sides where he appears dangerous, destructive, and terrible. Shivaism is expected in the Himalayan region and is mainly yogic. Some Hindu ascetics also worship him.

The 13th to 16th centuries were an excellent time for Shivaite ascetics and Natha yogis in northern India. They practiced Hatha yoga and various tantric rituals. Gorakhnatha is the most famous Natha yogi. He was a student of Matsyendranatha, a disciple of Siva. Through Hatha yoga, one could stop the body's decay and activate kundalini Shakti to create an immortal body leading to the Shiva state. According to Natha yogis, only Hatha yoga could lead to this condition; other religious paths were considered unnecessary.

About two percent of Hindus follow Shaktism and worship the goddess Shakti, the female power of the supreme divine principle. She is seen as the ultimate reality (Brahman), the creative force (Shakti), the matter in creation (Prakriti), the one who hides (Maya), and the savior. Shaktism has evolved from Shivaism. Many female figures were found during the excavations in the Indus Valley, although it is unclear what they represented. In the seventh century A.D., Shaktism was mentioned in the written traditions.

Female ideology also plays a central role in tantrism, whose concept is based on the belief that our external environment and bodies consist of both female and male aspects and that salvation comes through uniting this polarity. To achieve tantric salvation (sadhana), mantras, mudras, nyasa, and puja are used. Tantrism combines Jnana and Karma yoga. Knowledge ultimately saves a person, and action gives them experience of the ultimate reality. Kundalini yoga was developed as a separate branch of yoga within tantrism and is based on the goddess ideology of tantrism and Shaktism. The path of tantrism is the most effective for the world we live in today, the Kali era. Old techniques are more challenging to apply.

HINDUISM AND YOGA

In the 1920s, archaeological excavations along the Indus River uncovered the remains of two large cities, Mohenjo Daro and Harappa. Both yoga and Hinduism most likely originated from this era, when the Indus and Saraswati civilizations existed.

The excavations also uncovered fall stones, an essential symbol of the God Shiva, and signets, one of which depicted a person with animal horns sitting in a meditation position surrounded by four animals. Shiva is often called the master of animals, which may indicate that he was already being worshipped when the Indus culture flourished between 5,000 and 3,000 BC. Shiva is called the great yogi, suggesting that yoga originated from this time.

Modern technology has helped establish that the Saraswati River dried up sometime in the 30th century B.C. The river Saraswati is praised in the Rigveda, suggesting this sacred text must have come into being earlier. Yoga is mentioned in the Rigveda, indicating that it originated before the 30th century B.C.

Yoga is central to Hinduism and a physical and mental discipline to achieve spiritual salvation. Most people have experienced this part of Hinduism – both Hindus and non-Hindus. The original goal of yoga in the Hindu tradition is to reach salvation or enlightenment with the help of the body, using various physical and mental techniques. In the West, yoga has been chiefly used to strengthen the body and find peace. Like Hinduism, yoga is pluralistic, meaning many physical and mental exercises depend on your chosen tradition.

Traditions can define the concept of yoga in different ways. The most common translation among Hindus is "union," which refers to a union between body and soul. The Patanjali Yoga Sutras, one of the most essential texts in yoga, defines yoga chitta vritti nirodhah, or cessation of the activities of the mind.

Within the yoga traditions, the term yoga has five primary meanings:

1. A disciplined method of achieving a goal.

2. A technique for controlling the body.

3. A name for one of the six philosophical systems of Hinduism.

4. Combined with words such as Hatha, mantra, and laya, yoga refers to traditions focusing on specific yoga techniques.

5. Objectives for the practice of yoga.

Central to any tradition is breathing and breath control. Holding the breath is considered a ritual act in the Brahmanic tradition. Atharvaveda tells of breathing and its connection to the body's energies. The Chandogya Upanishad describes five different types of breathing: inner sound, and nadis.

YOGA AND BUDDHISM

Buddhism has its roots in Indian yoga and was, from its beginning, a form of yoga. Yoga teachers taught the Buddha himself, and his experiences became the basis of the Buddhist meditation doctrine. Buddhists and Hindu yoga are thus closely related and may have influenced each other for hundreds of years. Concepts such as nirodha / nirvana (cessation) and dukkha (suffering) are expected in both traditions. The Buddhist eight-fold path and Indian eight-fold yoga have many similarities. The big difference is that in Indian yoga, the body and breathing have a much greater significance. The most crucial goal in both traditions is to end avidya, false knowledge.

THE SCRIPTURES OF VEDA

Veda means knowledge, and the scriptures are divided into four parts (Samantha):

1. The Rigveda (roughly the 30th century B.C.) is the oldest part of the Vedic scriptures, where yoga and the Saraswati river are mentioned. These Vedas are recited hymns and serve as regulations for various rituals. Different yoga techniques were developed to strengthen the ability to concentrate to perform the ceremonies successfully.

2. The Samaveda are Vedas with sung hymns.

3. The Yajurveda are Vedas with ritual texts.

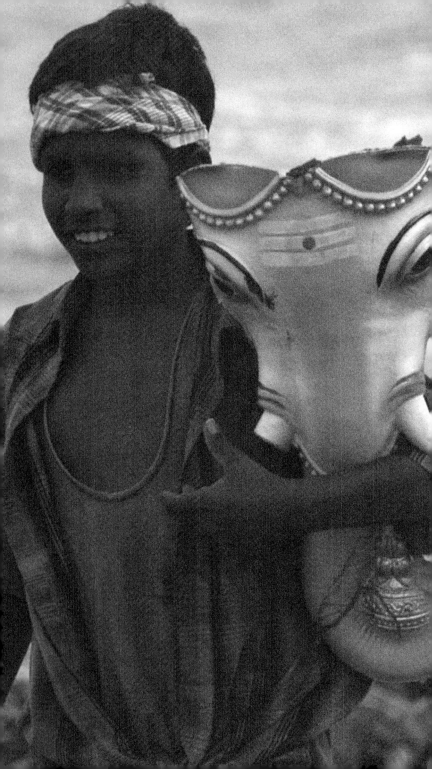

4. The Atharvaveda are Vedas with magic formulas.

According to the Vedic worldview, our world reflects the cosmic world. One can create a harmonious existence by maintaining the heavenly order on our planet. To get an inner picture of the cosmic order, followers use yoga techniques such as regulated breathing, mantra singing, and concentration exercises.

These four parts are the first part of the Vedas. Three additional texts are included:

1. Brahmana: comments on the vedas that explain the rituals of each samitha.

2. Aranyaka: "Forest books".

3. The Upanishads: The last part of the Vedas and often seen as the most important. This esoteric text describes the worldview in Vedanta, India's most famous philosophical system.

The Upanishads are based on four fundamental concepts:

1. The Brahman (world soul) is identical to the atman (the human soul), which means that the creative energy of the universe is similar to our inner self.

2. The realization that the unity of everything leads to spiritual enlightenment – moksha. This insight frees us from the cycle of rebirth.

3. The law of karma means that our thoughts and actions affect our future.

4. You are born according to your karma if you do not reach insight.

In the Katha, Svetasvarata, and Maitri Upanishads, you can find descriptions of yoga exercises and Samkhya concepts and performances, indicating that yoga has been associated with Samkhya from an early age.

"It is the highest state:
When the five sense organs
and the mind have calmed down,
and the intellect is immobile.
They call this control of the senses yoga.
Then he is free from disturbances,
for yoga is both origin and cessation."

(Katha-upanishad 6.10-11)

"By holding the body with its top three parts
right and getting the feelings and senses to
go in the heart, the sage crosses all
dangerous rivers with Brahman as a boat.

While controlling breathing and all movements, he should breathe through his nose
with manipulated breathing sounds, the
wise control his mind as he steers a chariot
drawn by wild horses.

In an even and clean place, free from pebbles,
fire, and sand, near running water, in one
location the mind finds attractive and to
which the eye does not react as ugly, in a
hidden area sheltered from the wind, he
should practice yoga."

(Svetasvatara-upanishad 2.8-2.10)

THE MAHABHARATA

Yoga is also mentioned in the Mahabharata, which belongs to the category of itihasa (history) and which is one of two great epic works in Hinduism, especially in Books 12 and 13, where yoga is described in close connection with Samkhya.

"WHAT YOGIS SEE IS THE SAME AS
THE FOLLOWERS OF SAMKHYA PERCEIVE.
HE IS A SAGE WHO SEES SAMKHYA AND YOGA AS THE
SAME."

(MAHABHARATA 12.293.30)

The Bhagavad Gita is a mythological work of poetry and the most crucial scripture in Bhakti yoga. This great epic belongs to the Mahabharata and was added about 700 AD. It is seen as a summary of the Upanishads. Here, Krishna is described as the master of yoga, which is seen as a disciplined method of achieving a goal. Three yoga paths are described – Jnana, Karma, and Bhakti, of which Bhakti is considered the highest.

"IT IS BETTER TO FOLLOW ONE'S DHARMA BADLY
THAN ANOTHER'S FLAWLESSLY."

(BHAGAVAD GITA 3.35)

"WHILE SITTING THERE,
HE SHOULD PRACTICE YOGA
TO CLEAR THE MIND,
KEEP THE MIND ATTACHED TO AN OBJECT,
AND RESTRAIN THE MIND
AND EMOTIONS ACTIVITY."

(BHAGAVAD GITA 6.12)

DIFFERENT YOGA PATHS

As said, yoga is a broad tradition with many branches and techniques. Down the ages, masters have developed various methods for spiritual enlightenment. There are no direct boundaries between the yoga paths, but everyone goes in some way into each. Within a yoga tradition, one can use many different techniques.

KARMA YOGA – THE WAY OF ACTION

Karma yoga is a way of action and is mainly suitable for outgoing people. It means working, performing social activities, and helping others without expecting anything. Karma yoga continues the Vedic sacrificial doctrine, where sacrifices were made to the gods. In the Bhagavad Gita, sacrificial acts mean one is loyal to the warning doctrine that they follow their dharma and the class they belong to.

Today, Karma yoga is more about selfless, moral action. The job itself is not the most important; one's attitude during its execution is. One's mood determines whether the activity or job is perceived as liberating or binding, painful and challenging. Whatever you choose to do, make sure you always do your best. If you can do the job better, you do it. One should not let negative thoughts, such as fear of criticism, hold one back. You should also feel free of your job but be prepared to leave it if necessary. Mahatma Gandhi are a famous Karma yogi.

BHAKTI YOGA – THE WAY OF DEDICATION

This path is suitable for people who are emotional with nature. One surrenders oneself to God through prayers, worship, and rituals, driven by the power of love and experiencing God as love itself. Being devoted and loving towards a personal god is considered to lead to salvation. Chanting and singing God's name is a central part of Bhakti yoga.

RAJA YOGA – THE WAY OF MEDITATION

Often called the royal way, Raja yoga involves the control of thoughts. One trains the mind through meditation and transforms mental and physical energy into spiritual energy. Raja yoga is also called Ashtanga yoga, which refers to "eight-step yoga," which should systematically lead to control of the mind. Meditation takes place by itself when the body and energy are under control and in harmony.

Ashtanga yoga's eight steps – the Yoga Sutras of Patanjali:

1. Yamas – five basic ideas about moral discipline, "do not do":
Ahimsa – do not use violence.
Sathyam – be authentic.
Brahmacharya – moderation, control over desire, chastity.
Asteya – do not steal.
Aparighara – do not be greedy.

2. Niyamas – five basic ideas about ethical action, "should do":
Saucha – external and internal cleanliness, such as thoughts, speech, and hygiene.
Santosha – contentment.
Tapas – restraint, self–discipline.
Swadhyaya – studies.
Ishvara pranidhana – the worship of God.

3. Asana – body position.
The lotus position. To be able to sit utterly immobile so as not to be distracted by the physical body during meditation.

4. *Pranayamas – controlled breathing.*
Controlled breathing to control the prana in the body, which calms the mind.

5. *Pratyahara – directs the sense organs inward.*
It calms the mind when not disturbed by the environment and external stimuli.

6. *Dharana – concentration.*
Concentration is achieved by focusing on an object.

7. *Dhyana – meditation.*
After a long period of concentration, meditation is achieved.

8. *Samadhi – ecstasy.*
Prolonged meditation leads to ecstasy. The yogi becomes at one with the object of meditation when the movements of the mind cease.

JNANA YOGA – THE WAY OF KNOWLEDGE
This path is the most challenging because it requires a strong will and sharp intellect. It is suitable for theoretically inclined people. A Jnana yogi understands the transient and the eternal in life by studying Vedanta, which belongs to the Upanishads, the last part of the Vedic scriptures. It is challenging to reach spiritual insight through theoretical knowledge; therefore, it is essential to practice other yoga paths as a preparation. Ramana Maharishi is a well-known Jnana yogi.

THE MANTRA
The mantra consists of words and syllables that carry a unique vibration and affect the mind and body in a positive and strengthening way.

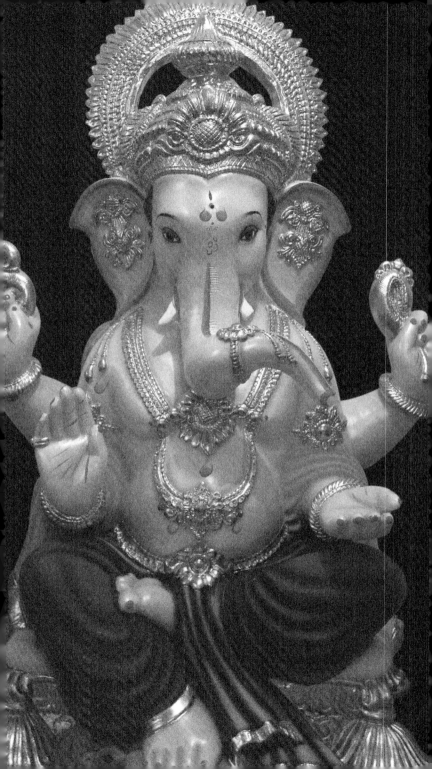

According to tradition, mantras have been used to reach a deeper plane of consciousness.

With mantra meditation, you calm your thoughts and mind. Repeating the same mantra repeatedly does not give the mind any new stimulus; instead, it allows the subconscious mind to wake up. Old thoughts and memories have an opportunity to come to the surface, and the subconscious mind can be purified from them. One looks more clearly at life and is no longer governed by old thought patterns. In the same way that asanas are meant to strengthen and purify the body, the mantra is meant to calm and "clean up" the mind.

In yoga, it is believed that everything in the universe consists of energy that vibrates differently. Mantras are high vibrations that should benefit and positively affect our bodies. When we recite or sing a mantra, we begin to vibrate at the same rate. Our palate has eighty-four meridian points that affect the pituitary gland, the pineal gland, and the brain's chemical balance. When we pronounce specific mantras, the tongue hits these meridian points, which can increase mental clarity and awareness.

Most often, one recites a mantra one hundred and eight times. Our physical and subtle body has seventy-two thousand energy channels called nadis. One hundred and eight meet at Hrit padma, the area around the Anahata chakra. By repeating a mantra one hundred and eight times, the whole physical and subtle body is permeated by its energy.

THE GAYATRI MANTRA

The gayatri mantra is said to be the oldest mantra, with its origins in the Rigveda Vedic scripture. It is sometimes called savitri because, in the mantra, one prays to Deva Savitr, the sun god who was worshipped during the Vedic period (the sun before sunrise is called savitri and after sunrise surya). The gayatri mantra is also found in other Hindu texts, such as the Bhagavad Gita, and is essential in Hindu traditions. It is taught to children when they turn eight years old.

The gayatri mantra is said to heal physically, mentally, and emotionally. It expands consciousness, promotes spiritual development, and develops intellectual potential, knowledge, and wisdom. It seems sattvic.

THE GAYATRI MANTRA

OM BHUR BHUVAHA SVAHA
TAT SAVITUR VARENYAM
BHARGO DEVASYA DHIMAHI
DHIYO YONAH PRACHODAYAT

"PRAISE TO THE SOURCE OF ALL THINGS.
IT IS DUE TO YOU THAT WE ATTAIN TRUE
HAPPINESS ON THE PLANES OF EARTH, ASTRAL,
CASUAL.
IT IS DUE TO YOUR TRANSCENDENT NATURE THAT
YOU ARE WORTHY OF BEING WORSHIPED AND
ADORED.
IGNITE US WITH YOUR ALL-PERVADING LIGHT."

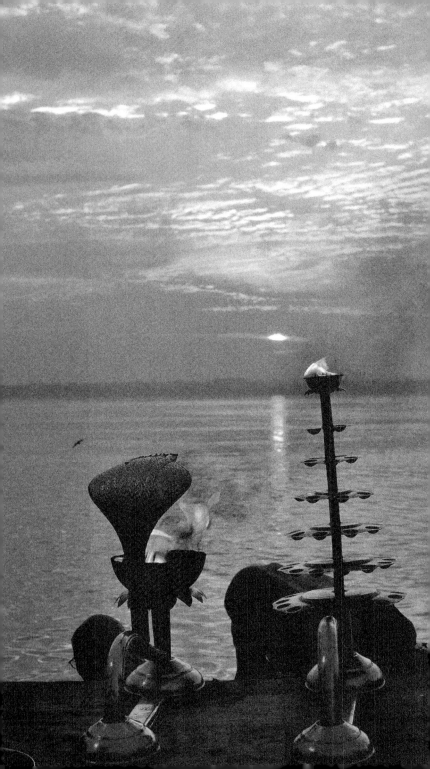

THE MAHAMRITYUNJAYA MANTRA

This mantra is also rooted in the Rigveda Vedic literature and is called the tryambakam mantra. It is dedicated to "the three-eyed," an epithet of Rudra, who was later characterized as Shiva.

The mahamrityunjaya mantra provides peace and protection. It is said to heal physically, mentally, and emotionally. It counteracts rajas.

THE MAHAMRITYUNJAYA MANTRA

OM TRIAMBAKAM YAJAMAHE
SUGANDHIM PUSHTI VARDANAM
URVARUKAMIVA BANDHANAN
MRITYOR MUKSHEEYA MAMRITAT

"SHELTER ME, THE THREE-EYED LORD SHIVA.
BLESS ME WITH HEALTH AND IMMORTALITY
AND SEVER ME FROM THE CLUTCHES OF DEATH,
EVEN AS A CUCUMBER IS CUT FROM ITS CREEPER."

THE INFLUENCE OF TANTRISM ON YOGA

During the post-classical period, it was primarily tantrism that influenced the yoga tradition.

According to tantrism, the human body's divine power (Kundalini Shakti) is inactive. This brings the physical body into focus for the ritual exercises, a new phenomenon in the spiritual history of India.

THE BHAGAVAD GITA

The Bhagavad Gita (the "Song of God") is the god Krishna's song. It is a mythological work in Sanskrit and an independent story in the great Mahabharata epic. In the Bhagavad Gita, a dialogue occurs between Krishna and Prince Arjuna just before the great battle of Kurukshetra. Arjuna faces a dilemma: his duty as a warrior is to follow his dharma and begin the war, but at the same time, he sees it as a terrible sin to kill the many great men, relatives, and gurus in the opponents' army. To accompany the prince through this challenging decision, Krishna teaches him various forms of yoga. The story takes place about five thousand years ago.

The Bhagavad Gita can be seen as a summary of the Upanishads. Each chapter ends with the Bhagavad Gita being called Upanishad.

Krishna says in Bhagavad Gita 3.3 that there have been two paths since ancient times:

Karma yoga – the way of action, to do one's duty without worrying about the outcome.

Jnana yoga – the way of knowledge, knowledge of the self (atman).

Other ways are variants of these.

Krishna shows his vishvarupa, his universal form, for Arjuna on the battlefield at Kurukshetra.

The Bhagavad Gita consists of eighteen chapters:

1. Arjuna lets Krishna pull his chariot to a place in the middle of the two armies. When Arjuna sees his relatives on the opposite side of Kurus, he loses motivation and decides not to fight.

2. Krishna explains to Arjuna that his concern about fighting against his relatives and gurus is unjustified because only the body can be killed, while the eternal self is immortal. Krishna reminds Arjuna to follow his dharma and wage war as a warrior.

3. Arjuna asks why he has to fight if knowledge is more important than action. Krishna emphasizes that the right way to act is to carry out one's duties for good without clinging to the results.

4. Krishna says he has lived through many births and always taught yoga to protect the righteous and annihilate the unrighteous. He emphasizes the importance of trusting a guru.

5. Arjuna asks Krishna if it is better to refrain from action or to perform actions. Krishna replies that both ways can be good, but that action, Karma yoga, is the highest.

6. Krishna describes the correct position of meditation and the process of achieving samadhi.

7. Krishna teaches the way of knowledge, Jnana yoga.

8. Krishna defines the terms Brahman, dharma, karma, atman, adhibhuta, and adhidaiva and explains how to remember him at the moment of death and attain a higher state.

9. Krishna describes panentheism, "all beings are in me," as a way of remembering him in all circumstances.

10. Krishna declares that he is the ultimate source of all material and spiritual worlds. Arjuna recognizes Krishna as the supreme being and quotes famous scholars who have done the same.

11. At Arjuna's request, Krishna demonstrates a theophany, its "universal form," Visvarupa: a terrifying creature that is turned in all directions at the same time, which spreads the radiation from a thousand suns around it, and which contains all other beings and all matter that exists.

12. Krishna describes the process of devotion, Bhakti yoga.

13. Krishna describes matter (Prakriti) and consciousness (Purusha).

14. Krishna talks about the three states, gunas, constituting all beings.

15. Krishna describes a symbolic tree, representing material existence, its roots in heaven, and its foliage on earth. He explains that this tree should be felled with the "axe of indifference" so that one can move on to a higher state.

16. Krishna describes the human traits of divine and demonic beings. He advises that the higher state can be achieved by renouncing lust, anger, and greed and distinguishing right actions from wrong deeds through buddhi and advice from scriptures, thereby acting right.

17. Krishna talks about the three variants of faith, knowledge, actions, and eating habits linked to the three gunas.

18. Krishna asks Arjuna to abandon all dharma and submit to him. He describes this as the ultimate and final perfection of life.

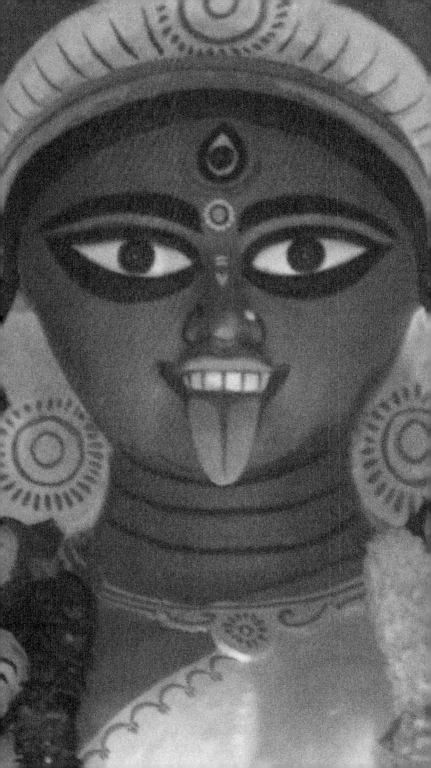

TANTRA
YOGA

TANTRA YOGA

TANTRA, MANTRA & YANTRA

The word tantra refers to those religious, literary works in which mysticism and magic play the leading role and form the ritual books belonging to the mysticism of later Hinduism.

Tantra books are intended to guide the use of magical and mysterious formulas and are often in the form of dialogues between Shiva and Durga. The word tantra comes from Sanskrit and combines the words tanoti and trayati, which can be translated as expansion and liberation. Tantra is about expanding the mind and releasing the dormant potential energy in man. Tantra sadhana – different tantric rituals – all evoke Kundalini Shakti differently.

To expand the mind, we must learn not to be controlled by our sensory experiences. When our senses and ego govern us, we categorize all our experiences into what we "like" and "do not like," which are called raga and dwesa. This categorization leads to suffering and inhibits our development and ability to see pure, actual knowledge. As we develop and expand the mind, we gradually build our intuitive ability, which is the source of accurate, eternal, and correct knowledge.

Daily, we perceive and take in our surroundings through our senses. If we instead learn to see, feel, listen, and turn the mind inwards, we can create an inner experience about ourselves and thus expand the mind. By releasing the energy (Shakti) and merging it with consciousness (Shiva), we create a homogeneous consciousness and experience Kundalini, which is the very purpose of tantra. The difference between tantra and most other spiritual and philosophical paths is that in tantra, you do not set up many rules that you have to live by.

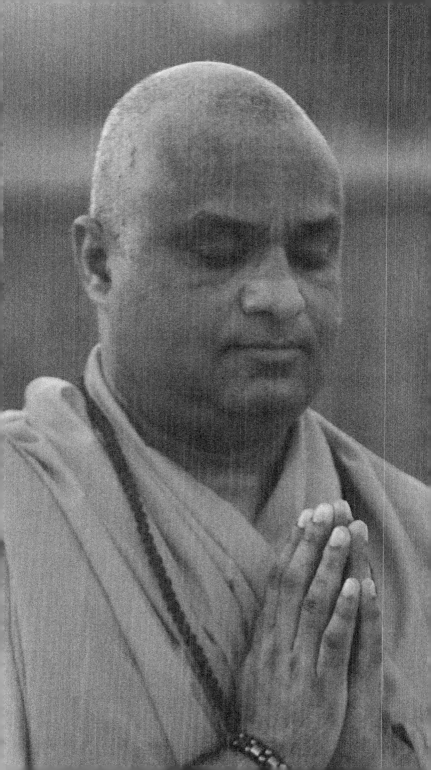

Everyone has an opportunity to develop, regardless of where they are. One can be sensualist or spiritualist, atheist or theist, poor or rich, strong or weak; the road is for everyone to discover. There are a total of sixty-four different tantras, and each one describes a different approach to mind control and expansion. Tantric techniques are often mistaken for being dirty and bizarre when alcohol, drugs, and sex are included in specific exercises and rituals. However, it is not used as a means of pleasure but to expand the mind.

Tantra describes Shakti, the subtle form of energy, as a coiled snake at the bottom of the body at the end of the spine, at the Mooladhara chakra. Shiva, the pure consciousness, is said to have its seat on top of the head in the Sahasrara chakra. To awaken the Kundalini energy, which in most people is dormant, one must first increase the flow and amount of prana, the vital energy down to the Mooladhara chakra. Then, Kundalini Shakti can be directed up to the Sahasrara chakra. On its way up the spine, Kundalini Shakti passes six chakras or energy pools. When Kundalini Shakti rises, they are charged with energy. The chakras act as nodes for our nadis energy channels, which vibrate at different intensities. Chakras carry dormant creative forces partially evident in our daily lives and whose full potential can only emerge when Kundalini Shakti have passed through them on their way up to Shiva.

Tantric exercises are divided into three steps in the form of upasana or worship:

Shuddhi – purification of the gross, subtle and psychic elements or tattwas.

Sthiti – enlightenment by concentration achieved by purifying the elements.

Arpana – insight into the cosmic consciousness.

Tantric exercises can be easily distinguished from other non-tantric exercises by the sacred formulas, symbols, and rituals. We want to attract higher subtle forces and our inner forces through worship and traditions. Tattwa shuddhi is one of the tantric rituals.

FIRST STEP – CLEANING THE ELEMENT

One of the first introductory tantric rituals is tattwa shuddhi, also known as bhuta shuddhi, which aims to purify our elements.
In tantra, tattwa / bhuta shuddhi transforms the pranic flow from our elements so it returns to the original unmanifested form – Shakti. As long as the prana flows in our external organs and is fixed in our elements, our consciousness will be limited to the external world. The energy / consciousness is thus improved and modified to our physical body through our elements. By releasing it, we can also make it expand.

The first step towards expansion is purifying our basic physical, mental, psychic, and pranic structures. In yoga, various purifying techniques are aimed at this: prana shuddhi, nadi shuddhi, vak shuddhi, manas shuddhi, etc. But the practice of tattwa / bhuta shuddhi, according to the ancient tantras, is comprehensive. The techniques used in tattwa shuddhi are:

Nyasa – concentration on the body.

Prana prathishta – is the placement of life and prana in the mandala.

Panchopchara – five things sacrificed in the worship of tattwan.

Japa – mantra repetition.

In many ancient tantric texts, tattwa shuddhi is described as an essential technique to move development forward and gain greater insight. Tattwa shuddhi strengthens our personal experiences of energy and pure consciousness. It is not enough to "know" intellectually that all matter originates in pure consciousness; it must be experienced. Personal experience is the core of tantra and can be made possible with the help of tattwa shuddhi.

By focusing on tattwa yantras, we increase the prana in the body and affect each chakra. Each tattwa is tied to a chakra. Charging each chakra prepares the awakening of the Kundalini Shakti and facilitates its path up to the Sahasrara chakra. Tattwa shuddhi also develops our ability to concentrate (dharana), which leads to spontaneous meditation (dhyana), which in turn leads to awareness of the subtle essence behind matter and form (tattwa jnana).

BRIEF DESCRIPTION OF TATTWA SHUDDHI
With the help of meditation and self-reflection, the elements that make up the mind and body are purified and transformed. Tattwa shuddhi is a dynamic form of meditation and self-reflection. It is not a passive form where you must focus on the same symbol for a long time. During the implementation of tattwa shuddhi, one quickly deepens the mind by creating images of tattwa yantras (geometric images of the elements), Papa Purusha (the sinful man), and the mandala of Prana Shakti (the form of the creative energy).

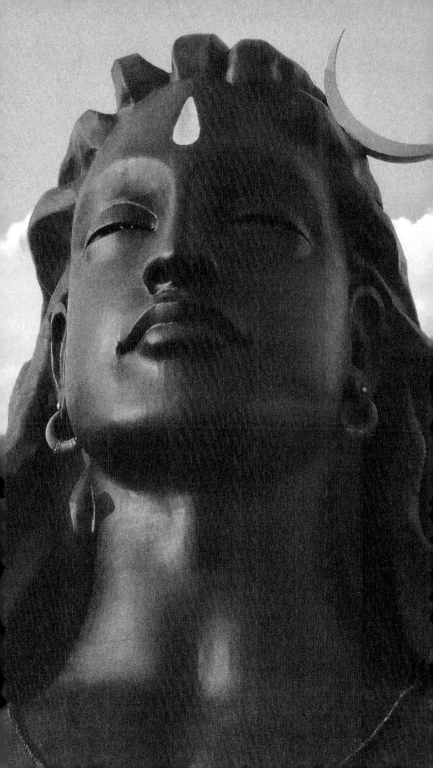

You start the exercise by creating a mental image of the elements and their respective yantra in the body. You witness how the elements are born from each other, and you thus sink deeper into yourself. When one discovers the universal cosmic energy within, one uses the power to heal inner imbalances. With the help of a higher state of consciousness and a stronger mind, it is easier to heal imbalances. After this, an internal image of the elements is again created, but in reverse order. Towards the end, one visualizes an image of prana shakti, the energy manifested through the elements. Finally, apply bhasma or ash to the body. Tattwa shuddhi can be used to enter a meditative state or as a complete sadhana.

It would help if you had practiced Hatha yoga and ajapa japa for a long time to get the most out of the exercise. The mind and body must be in good condition. You must be able to sit still for a long time without the mind being disturbed by the surroundings. Just before the exercise, it is a crucial preparation to turn the mind inward, which is best done with the help of pranayamas and trataka. You should also have a good knowledge of the location of the chakras in the body and how the prana moves along the sushumna. If you are ill, you should wait until you have recovered before practicing tattwa shuddhi.

CLEANING PROCESS
Tattwa shuddhi is a process that cleanses the elements of our body and purifies the senses connected to those elements. The sense of hearing is purified using mantra repetition; the sight by observing yantras and mandalas; the feeling and our tactile nerves by applying bhasma or ash to the body; the sense of smell by breathing exercises; and the sense of taste by eating sattvic food or by fasting.

Tattwa shuddhi cleanses not only our physical body but also the layers of our bodies. In addition to our physical body, we have several other bodies relating to the invisible parts of the mind that are affected by samskaras (latent impressions), which create sankalpa and vikalpa (thoughts / counter-thoughts) in our conscious mind.

Imbalances in the various bodies manifest themselves in the form of anxiety, distress, depression, and fear. We often find it difficult to cure these conditions in the same way as physical illnesses. In the long run, these imbalances affect our life and our personality. Our body is an extension of our mind, and each affects the other. Since the mind controls our body and its functions, it is as essential to purify your mental mind as your physical body.

In tantra, it is said that no action or thought is unclean or wrong—the unclean lies in false perception and judgment. Through the sadhana, we can come to an understanding of this and thus fight it. Without purifying the subtle levels of the mind, reaching higher levels of consciousness is impossible. An unclean mind cannot focus or concentrate. By harmonizing the flow of prana in the body, separating the intellect and ego from the consciousness, one can purify the different levels of the mind so that one becomes the experiencer and the witness simultaneously.

CLEANING OF THE ELEMENT
Tattwa shuddhi is a unique technique because it purifies the whole person from the coarsest layers to the most subtle. The first step in the cleansing process is to wash and cleanse the physical body, apply bhasma or ash, and fast and control food intake. Tantra emphasizes the importance of doing all everyday chores with awareness and presence.

Everything you do, how you sit, walk, talk, wash, etc., reflects your state of mind. Tattwa shuddhi is thus a purification process that covers all twenty-four hours of the day. However, the first step in physical purity is more about discipline than raising awareness.

The second step in the process purifies the subtle levels. You use your mind and prana. Internal forces are aroused and controlled by the elements. By refining the elements, the energy increases so that they can vibrate harmoniously, which creates a balance that leads to an increased inner awareness. By repeating the bija mantra and visualizing the yantra of each tattwa, one can dissolve deeply rooted samskaras and archetypes that prevent us from experiencing infinite consciousness.

PRANA SHAKTI

In our body, the prana moves in a specific pattern, meaning vibrations are created at different frequency levels. The vibrational frequencies build up our physical body and our subtle organs. We can see and feel the bodily organs and their constituents while the delicate organs are experienced. In tantra and yoga, these delicate organs are chakras, nadis, Kundalini Shakti, chitta Shakti, prana vayu and pancha tattwa.

The prana exists in the microcosm and macrocosm. Without it, we would not function or exist. We would not have the ability to see, hear, or move. Most of us have too little flow of prana in our body, which leads to fatigue and exhaustion.

The cosmic prana in our body is represented by Kundalini Shakti, which has its seat in the Mooladhara chakra. When its full potential is awakened, it rises along the central nervous system of our physical body, which in our pranic body is called the sushumna nadi. Kundalini Shakti also manifests itself in our more significant six chakras.

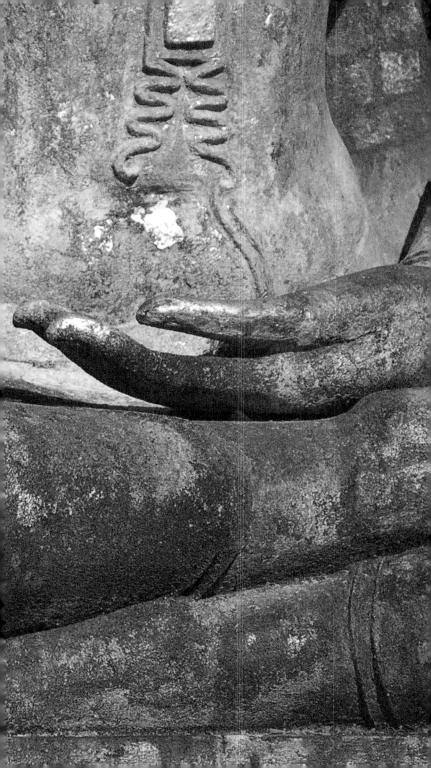

Each chakra consists of one element. In Mooladhara there are elements of the earth – prithvi tattwa; in Swadhisthana elements of water – apas tattwa; in Manipura elements of fire – agni tattwa; in Anahata elements of air – vayu tattwa; and in Vishuddhi elements of ether or space – akasha tattwa. The element that controls the chakra reveals the frequency at which the chakra vibrates. Our entire consciousness, thoughts, and actions are governed by the degree of activity of the chakra. Pingala nadi supplies chakras with energy, and Kundalini Shakti activates them to their full potential. When our chakras are only partially activated, we become limited in acting and experiencing. In tattwa shuddhi, we affect each chakra directly by concentrating on each tattwa.

MANDALA BY PRANA SHAKTI

In tantra, there is a tradition of symbolizing the various aspects of man in the form of mandalas. Mandalas represent the human subconscious and unconscious mind. Concentrating on these images can relax samskaras or archetypes that stand in the way of our creativity and knowledge. In tattwa shuddhi sadhana, a picture of prana Shakti is created as a beautiful goddess who has a powerful effect on us.

Prana Shakti, as a goddess, is red. Red is a base color that stands for raja guna. The color also symbolizes the dynamic quality of prana. Her six arms represent the efficiency she has in everything she undertakes. She holds a tool in each hand that illustrates different aspects of human existence. Her three eyes stand for prophecy, and the lotus flower she sits on for developing powers and siddhis.

ANTAH KARANA

Antah karana is man's inner tool and consists of four parts: buddhi *(intellect), ahamkara (ego), manas (thoughts and counter-thoughts), and chitta (memory). According to tantra and yoga, these four are the core of consciousness, which acts from the outside. Antah karana is unique and can only be found in humans. In lower life forms (animals and plant species), antah karana exists only as a precursor. Plants and animals act instinctively, not based on ego, intellect, or thoughts. Antah karana is what sets man apart from other species.*

Through antah karana, the human consciousness interprets, classifies and perceives everything that concerns the past, present and future. It is a recipient who receives and sends out impressions. In antah karana, in addition to the knowledge of this life and what happens here, there is also the knowledge of the universe and cosmos. This knowledge is often unmanifested and dormant in humans. Refining the frequency of antah karana is part of human evolution.

Antah karana is an instrument built up through all our incarnations. It carries all the impressions of our past lives. Antah karana determines the individual's future actions based on previous experiences and knowledge. These experiences and expertise are often unconscious unless we develop our inner vision and experience of the cosmos. Through tantric techniques, we can learn to see and control antah karana, which is part of our evolution.

DIMENSIONS OF THE MIND

In yoga, the mind is divided into four parts: jagriti (conscious mind), swapana (unconscious mind), sushpati (subconscious mind) and turya (our transcendental mind). In modern psychology, only the first three are mentioned.

Antah karana acts based on the conscious, subconscious, and uncons-
cious mind. Manas and chitta, which are part of the conscious and
subconscious mind, control thoughts and actions on the conscious and
subconscious plane. Buddhi and ahamkara constantly exist to varying
degrees in the conscious, subconscious, and unconscious mind. Since
all of these have arisen from the same principle, Shakti, they influence
each other intensively.

The three gunas, sattva, rajas, and tamas, lay the foundation for antah
karana. These three cosmic principles significantly influence manas,
chitta, and buddhi and thus affect our experiences. The fourth sense,
turya, is unaffected by the interplay between the three gunas. Turya
can only be developed by refining antah karana through sadhana. In
tattwa shuddhi, we learn to perceive antah karana and use its full
potential for further spiritual development.

BUDDHI

Buddhi is the principle that most closely resembles pure consciousness.
It motivates us to follow our dharma. Sattvic buddhi is characterized
by wisdom, happiness, perseverance, calm, self-control and discernme-
nt. Under the influence of rajas, some defects occur, which means that
the ability to distinguish deteriorates, and even actions are affected
by wrong knowledge and avidya. A tamasic buddhi acts under the
ego, which is judgmental and permeated by misinterpretations of the
outside world. In tattwa shuddhi, the principle of buddhi is meditated
on sattvic. It removes the qualities of rajas and tamas that stand in the
way of sattvic buddhi.

AHAMKARA

Aham means "I," and ahamkara is the ego or what one experiences as the "self." The ego is the core of individualism, which makes us identify with matter. Ahamkara is very subtle. At the same time as the ego binds man to objective experiences, it is the core that must be opened to experience unity. Without the ego, man would not be aware of his existence. On the conscious plane, the ego acts through our physical body, senses, and mind. On the subconscious plane, it works through our astral body and dreams. During deep sleep, the ego withdraws, while during meditation, it functions as the inner consciousness.

Sattvic ahamkara acts as a catalyst for self-realization. Ahamkara usually takes up the comrades and underlying experiences from the subconscious mind, but in a sattvic state, this stops. Rajasic ahamkara raises the identification with the "self," leading to restlessness and a constant need to do something. A tamasic ahamkara strengthens painful and negative samskaras, which causes fear and doubt. Through tattwa shuddhi, we can see how the ego works and thus stop identifying with it.

MANAS AND CHITTA
Manas and chitta represent the external mind: thoughts in our waking state and during dreams. Chitta is the core of all experiences in the form of samskaras, archetypes, and memories. Manas, i.e., our thoughts, are chitta's tools that coexist and by which archetypes and memories are expressed. Manas and chitta do not work individually but are influenced by both buddhi and ahamkara. Our manas are steady, focused, and concentrated in a sattvic state. Our senses are activated under the influence of rajas, creating an imbalance in our intellect. Tamasic manas make the intellect and the senses sluggish and inactive.

When chitta is in a sattvic state, our senses are withdrawn so that consciousness remains undisturbed. Under the influence of rajas, rajasic awakened samskaras in chitta in the form of vikalpa (fantasy) and viparayaya (wrong knowledge). In that state, chitta contains cohabitation, knowledge and ignorance, passion and freedom. When tamas prevail in chitta, unwanted samskaras will emerge as vasanas (deep-rooted desires).

The coexistence of a negative nature can only be eliminated through reflection, dharana, and dhyana. Tattwa shuddhi helps us enter meditation, which aims to liberate the consciousness. Only then can we reflect on the structure of the elements and influence them.

PANCHA TATTWA – THE FIVE ELEMENTS

All matter comprises five elements, akasha, vayu, agni, apas and prithvi. The elements lay the foundation for the creation and make it last. The elements affect every aspect of our lives, thoughts, and actions. In yoga, it is essential to learn how these elements work to be able to control and influence them and our lives. In tantric texts, the science behind the elements is described.

The elements form a chain where they are born from each other. Akasha is the first element of the process. Akasha consists of subtle matter and energy, which rests in consciousness. When the energy in akasha begins to vibrate, movement is created, and vayu tattwa takes shape. Vayu stands for the movement that permeates everything. The intense movement creates heat, which causes the next element in the joint (agni) to be made. Agni tattwa has a slower vibration than vayu. It allows the heat to cool down and form apas and water elements. The vibration and movement of the apas are minimal. The last element,

*prithvi, occurs when the movement / vibration is further reduced. Apas
solidify and become the elements of the earth. The elements should
extend pure consciousness, not separate existing parts.*

*During evolution, tattwas have been further developed through tan-
matras. Tanmatra is the quality through which tattwas are perceived.
Akasha is perceived through shaba tanmatra (sound), vayu through
sparsha tanmatra (feeling), agni through roopa tanmatra (vision), apas
through rasa tanmatra (taste) and prithvi through gandha tanmatra
(smell). We are created from the roughest form of the elements when
we are born. In tattwa shuddhi, we have an experience of the elements
in their subtle form to develop spiritually.*

*The Patanjali Yoga Sutras state that each element consists of five
different characters. To take control of the elements, one must practice
samyama, a combination of concentration, meditation, and samadhi.
Patanjali called this bhuta jaya "knowledge of the elements." The first
character of the five elements is the rough form related to experiences
we take through our senses: sound, touch, form, taste, and smell. The
second character relates to the quality of the elements:*

- *The liquid property of water.*
- *The heat of the fire.*
- *The movement of air.*
- *The space of ether.*

*The third character is the subtle form of tanmatras. Here, tattwas are
experienced in quiet sounds, sensations, form, smell and taste and are
often called mental visions. The fourth aspect of the elements relates to
the three gunas (sattva, rajas, and tamas), which are an essential part*

of the elements. One should strive to transform the qualities of rajasic and tamasic into more sattvic to develop spiritually. Tattwa shuddhi enables this change. The fifth aspect of the elements is called artha-vattwa, which stands for the actual goal of the elements. The scriptures describe that it is for the liberation and enjoyment of consciousness from matter that the elements have developed.

The elements are characterized by shaba (sound) and warn (color) and are created by the vibration in the component. The color refers to the energy frequency of the element. Akasha is black, as the vibration is minimal. Vayu vibrates in the frequency of blue, agni in red, apas in white and prithvi in yellow. The second manifestation of the energy of the elements is sound in the form of bija mantras. Bija mantra for akasha is Ham, for vayu – Yam, agni – Ram, apas – Vam and prithvi – Lam.

Sound and color together build the form of energy. Akasha is experien-ced as a circle, vayu as a hexagon, agni as an inverted triangle, apas as a horizontal crescent moon and prithvi as a yellow square.

AKASHA TATTWA – the element of space.
Akasha can be described as the space or emptiness between two objects or matter. Akasha is the most subtle of all the elements and is almost motionless. It stands for the whole spectrum of sounds, from the rough to the quiet, and acts as a carrier for the sound. The vibration of the element is so subtle that it cannot be experienced with external senses. It is said that ether moves at a higher speed than sound. Akasha tattwa is boundless and permeates the entire cosmos; therefore, it has the shape of a circle. It is not of matter as we know it and cannot be expe-rienced physically. Tattwa jnanis has discovered akasha by refining the

rough mind. Because of this quality, tantra has described the element as mental (not physical) and the "space of the mind" behind closed eyes, called chidakasha. Tattwa akasha stands for the space in the body between our organs. On a mental level, tattwa akasha controls man's emotions and passions. The best time for meditation and concentration is when akasha flows in the body, which happens about five minutes every hour. The element has its seat on top of the head. Mentally, it relates to our unconscious mind, and its psychic centers are the Vishuddhi chakra. The spiritual experience created by the element is jnana loka and anandamaya kosha.

VAYU TATTWA – the element of air.

Vayu can be translated as air. The element is gray-blue and is symbolized by a hexagon. Vayu stands for kinetic energy in all its forms: electrical, chemical, vital, and prana. Its quality is movement, and it controls all movement qualities in the body, including prana, apana, samana, udana, and vyana. Vayu is responsible for our ability to experience physical touch. When we develop the mind for touch, we can experience the feeling of energy in us and around us. Even vayu is physically invisible. The element can be described as "energy in motion." Movement creates change, which means this element can cause stability and instability in humans and the environment. Vayu has its seat between the heart and the eyebrows. Mentally, the element relates to the subconscious mind. Its psychic center is the Anahata chakra. The spiritual experience of vayu is maha loka and vijnamaya kosha, our intuitive body.

AGNI TATTWA – the element of fire.

Agni or fire is called tejas, meaning "to sharpen." The element is primarily energy and is experienced as light. With the help of light, we

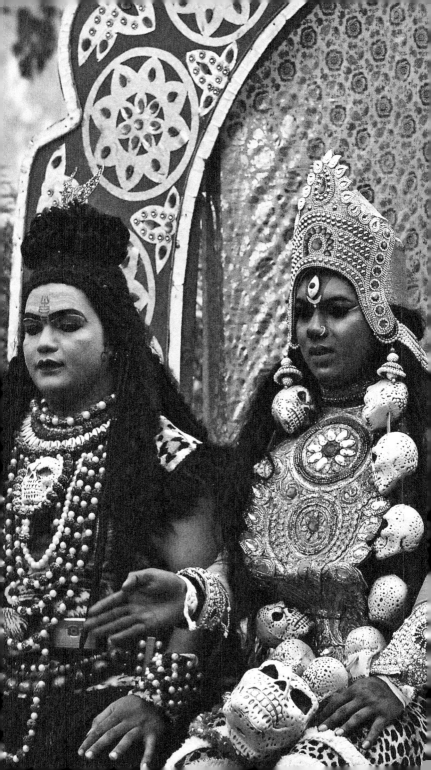

can see the shape. The sense organ that agni relates to is the eye, which allows us to see. Form or matter is the core of the emergence of our ego. The ego identifies with form, which leads to attachment to things. Agni tattwa is thus not only the first manifestation of the form and the stage when ahamkara begins to grow. The element wears the color red, which indicates fire and heat. The yantra is a red triangle. Agni is often called the "devouring force" and stands for instability. The power of fire is destructive but can be seen as a catalyst for change, development, and evolution. In our physical body, tattwa agni regulates our digestive fire, appetite, thirst, and sleep. It has its place between the heart and the navel. Its psychic centers are the Manipura chakra. The spiritual experience of the element is swar loka and manomaya kosha, our mental / thought body.

APAS TATTWA – the element of water.

Apas can be described as a large amount of intensively active matter that has emerged from agni tattwa. It is a matter that is not yet coherent, as the molecules and atoms are in great chaos. The universe is said to take the form of tattwa apas before it appears. Yantra, for the element, is a horizontal crescent surrounded by water. Our body can see apas through blood, mucus, bile, and lymph fluid as it controls our body fluids. The element affects our thoughts related to ourselves and worldly things. The apas has its seat between the navel and the knees. Mentally, it relates to our subconscious and conscious mind. Its psychic centers are the Swadhisthana chakra. The spiritual experience of tattwa apas is bhuvar loka and pranamaya kosha, our energy body.

PRITHVI TATTWA – the element of earth.

The last tattwa is prithvi, or bhumi, "to be". In prithvi, the motion of the particles has stopped almost completely. Energy has become matter in solid, liquid, or gas form. This element bears the yellow color, and the yantra is a yellow square. It has the qualities of firmness, weight, and cohesion. Our physical body can see this through bones and other organs. Since prithvi has emerged from all the other elements, it has all the qualities, but smell is the dominant quality. The component creates stability physically, mentally, and in our environment and stands for the material. It has its physical place between our toes and knees. Mentally, it relates to the conscious and subconscious mind. Its psychic center is the Mooladhara chakra. The spiritual experience of prithvi tattwa is bhu loka and annamaya kosha, our physical body.

TATTWAS AND KOSHAS

The elements build up layers that are called koshas in yoga. Man is said to have five layers, all of which vibrate differently and relate to different levels of consciousness. The first and coarsest layer is called annamaya kosha; our body is made of food. Pranamaya kosha is the layer of prana, manomaya kosha is the layer of thoughts, vijnamaya kosha is the layer of intuition, and the last layer is the layer of body bliss, anandamaya kosha.

These subtle layers of man can only be affected with the help of yoga, tantra, and other spiritual exercises. In tattwa shuddhi, annamaya kosha and pranamaya kosha are affected by controlling respiration and increasing the flow of prana. Manomaya kosha is affected by concentration. Vijnamaya kosha is aroused by concentration on tattwa yantras. There is no direct exercise to influence anandamaya kosha. Working with the other four layers of bodies is necessary to experience anandamaya kosha.

Experiences of color, light, and smell during tattwa shuddhi are experiences of our subtle bodies.

Koshas are also linked to seven planes of consciousness. These are called lokas. Each loka relates to a plane of existence through which consciousness develops. The elements influence each loka, and through tattwa shuddhi, we also influence these.

TATTWAS AND BREATHING

Elements such as chitta Shakti, prana Shakti and atma Shakti are manifested in our physical body. These act in the body and mind through our energy channels, nadis or breathing (swara). Swara and nadi mean flow. Nadi is the flow of Shakti in our subtle body while swara shastra is the flow of our breathing in nadis. Swara shastra is thus the science behind the flow of breathing and nadis. The three Shakti that flow in our breath are channeled through three main nadis in the body (ida, pingala and sushumna). It is said that we have about seventy-two thousand nadis in the body. Ida, pingala, and sushumna are responsible for the psychosomatic and spiritual parts of the body, mind, and consciousness.

Chitta Shakti, the power of ida nadi, is the vital and mental energy that controls all our functions regarding thoughts, mind, and chitta. All mental activity is the result of the flow of ida. This flow is connected to our left nostril and affects the right side of the brain. It is also called chandra swara and relates to the negative aspect of the energy in the body.

Prana Shakti flows through the pingala nadi. It is the vital life energy and relates to the positive aspect of it. Prana Shakti controls all physical *activity. The flow of pingala nadi is connected to our right nostril and affects the left side of the cerebral hemisphere. It is also called surya swara. Atma Shakti is channeled through sushumna nadi—Pranan's central passage for spiritual consciousness. Sushumna is neutral energy active when breathing flows through both nostrils simultaneously. This condition affects the activity of the dormant parts of the brain. In our physical body, these three nadis relate to the parasympathetic (ida), sympathetic (pingala) and autonomic (sushumna) nervous systems. In most people, sushumna is closed for most of their lives, meaning ida and pingala control them. Through yogic and tantric exercises, one can open up sushumna nadi.*

These three aspects of energy manifest in our breathing cycles. The flow lasts about an hour in each nostril. When the flow changes, the sushumna is open for a few seconds. In our flow of swara, the elements are included. Each element has a specific pranic frequency and affects various bodily functions. Tattwas cause the swara to flow in different directions and affect ida, pingala and sushumna. Ida and pingala nadi channel shakti to the chakras in the body and affect their vibration. The elements also affect the chakras in the body through breathing. Each chakra is dominated by one element – Mooladhara by the earth element, Swadhisthana by the water element, Manipura by the fire element, Anahata by the air element, and Vishuddhi by the air element. Just as breathing affects our mental, physical, and spiritual existence, so do the elements, through their different character, affect our state of mind, body, and consciousness.

Through various tantric and yogic techniques, it is possible to practice the feeling for which tattwa is active in the swara for the moment. A tattwa yogi can assess his physical, mental, emotional and spiritual condition in this way. Examples of exercises that practice the ability are trataka on tattwa yantras and sensations of the elements (color and shape) during the performance of naumukhi mudra, yoni mudra or shanmukhi mudra. The last-mentioned exercises practice our knowledge and experience of the elements as they work. You close the gates for external perception and simultaneously open up to the inner experience of color, sound, smell, and form.

MANTRA, YANTRA & MANDALA

The theory and philosophy behind tantra are closely intertwined with mantra, yantra, and mandala. Tantra is a philosophical and practical science whose sublime theories become effective through mantra, yantra, and mandala. The unique thing about tantra is that there is always an explanation and valuable exercise for each philosophy or theory. Mantra, yantra and mandala are used in all tantric exercises, also within tattwa shuddhi.

MANDALA

The word mandala means circle, and in Hindu and Buddhist rituals, it refers to a figure drawn on the ground or painted on a table that symbolizes the cosmic and celestial regions. A mandala is a meditation figure constructed of circles and shapes. Correctly depicted and properly inaugurated, it becomes a concentration of occult energy, which attracts hidden forces and emits rays like a talisman. Within the boundaries of the mandala circle, other geometric figures are drawn: smaller squares, triangles, and circles that divide it all into sacred zones.

To create a mandala, one must be able to see into oneself. Not by thinking – but by vision, as clearly and distinctly as with open eyes. The more precise the inner vision, the more influential the created man-

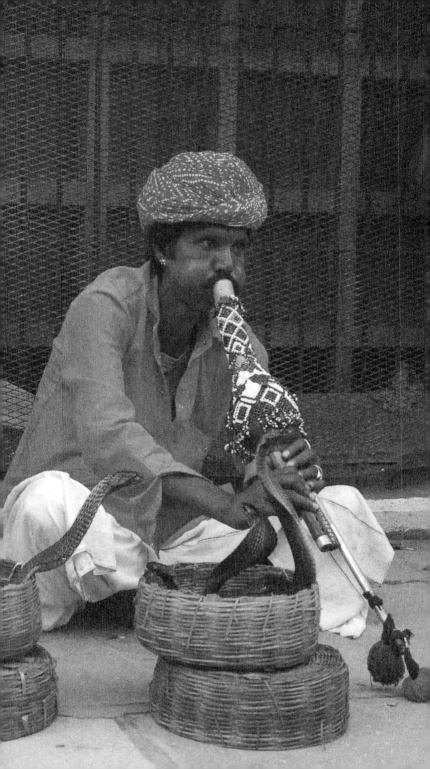

dala. The principle behind a mandala is that it exists in the form of a circle. The circle stands for the basic shape behind everything. Anything can shape a mandala, a tree, a house, a car, an animal, or a human being. Even the body is a mandala. To create a mandala that carries strength and power, one must be able to create an exact copy of the inner vision. A mandala is the essence of an object experienced by someone who has refined the inner eye, an inner cosmic image of which everyone can partake. The level of consciousness lays the foundation for what the mandala will look like. All forms of art, sculpture, and architecture are from the beginning mandala's given form.

In tantra, mandalas are also depicted as illustrated images of divine forces. A human form of the sacred makes it easier for the rough mind of man to understand and experience the power within when the ability to visualize is weak. The symbolism and structure behind the images of deities are intended to awaken the equivalent in the individual's consciousness. By concentrating on mandalas, deeply rooted samskaras are awakened within.

Perhaps the most talked about mandala created in tantra is maithuna kriya. Maithuna kriya forms a mandala that has corresponding yantras and mantras. The erotic sculptures of the Khajuraho Temple in Orissa are based on the tantric belief that maithuna is intended to awaken man's divine forces. The man represents Shiva, the physical energy, and the woman, Shakti, the mental energy. Mandalas are created as a force field or energy circle through their exoteric and esoteric union. Linga and yoni mandala are also symbols of this higher union. Man and woman physically unite to re-experience the unity from which they were created. This union is an inner experience in the same way as the spiritual experience.

YANTRA

*A yantra is an abstract mathematical image of an inner vision. Be-
hind each rough shape is a subtle shape, which the yantra represents.
Everything in nature can be experienced in its original form (yantra).
It carries an inherent energy just like everything else in creation. By
visualizing and concentrating on the yantra, one can awaken the
corresponding energy in oneself. The yantra comprises the primary and
original shapes: a bindu / dot, a circle, a square, and a triangle. Bindu
is the point from which everything has been created and to which everything will return; it is the process of creation and dissolution. It also
represents the union between Shiva and Shakti. Bindu is also found
in our body, on the top of the back of the head, and is called Bindu
visarga. During meditation, one uses the outer Bindu as a yantra to
experience the contraction of time and space in bindu in the physical
body. The triangle stands for the first shape that comes out of creation
and is also known as the moola tricona (spelling should be trikona in
English). Upside down, it stands for Prakriti (creation), and with the
tip facing upwards, it stands for Purusha (consciousness). The circle
represents the cycle of timelessness where neither the beginning nor
the end exists, only eternity. It symbolizes the process of birth, life, and
death. The square is the base on which the yantra rests and represents
the physical, earthly world that must be refined.*

*Yantras create a path from the outer to our inner. They are essential
for our continued spiritual evolution: they strengthen our creative and
intuitive sides and spiritual experiences. In tattwa shuddhi, one uses
yantra created from the four primary forms.*

MANTRA

In the same way that every thought has an equivalent in the form of an image, every image also has an equivalent in sound, nada, or vibration. These sounds are called mantras. Mantra means "contemplating what leads to liberation." Nada is one of the first manifestations of creation, the form. In Indian philosophy, it is believed that the first sound of creation was the sound of "Om," which is the cosmic mantra. Mandukyo Upanishad describes how the mantra affects and expands different levels of consciousness. "Om" is made up of three syllables, "A", "U", and "M", which all vibrate at different frequencies, which affect the consciousness in different ways. When you repeat "Om," you raise awareness to the same frequency as the mantra. It applies to all mantras.

Nada consists of four frequencies: para (cosmic), pashyanti (temporary), madhyama (subtle) and vaikhari (rough) and correspond to the four frequency levels that "Om" carries: consciously, unconsciously, subconsciously and turya. The entire Sanskrit alphabet consists of mantras. In Sanskrit, the letters are not called letters but akshara, which means imperishable. Each akshara can be used as a mantra. Therefore, it is said that only by reading Vedas can one achieve liberation.

The most potent form of the mantra is the bija mantra. Bija means seed and is the sound from which all other mantras are derived. The Bija mantra is a powerful, concentrated energy attributed to different levels of consciousness. In tattwa shuddhi, bija mantras related to the five elements are used. Even in tantra, it is known that each physical body part has a mantra to which it corresponds. These mantras are used in nyasa to transform the physical body into a container for more extraordinary powers, which is aroused by tattwa shuddhi and other esoteric techniques.

Breathing has its mantra created by inhaling (So) and exhaling (Ham) and is known as the ajapa japa mantra. In the Upanishads, it is said that this mantra is powerful enough in itself to awaken Kundalini Shakti and expand consciousness. In the introduction to tattwa shuddhi, the mantra So Ham creates a sense of belonging to the universal consciousness.

By repeating the mantra, you raise the consciousness, and by concentrating on a yantra, you focus the consciousness to a point. At a level of consciousness, the inner experience manifests as a thought or emotion; at a higher level, it becomes an inner vision or mandala. It becomes a yantra later manifested as sound, nada, or mantra when you go deeper. When the mind functions under lower and coarser energy frequencies, it becomes static, sluggish, slow, and tamasic. When you make the energy more subtle through mantra, yantra, and mandala, the state of mind changes from tamasic to becoming rajasic and finally sattvic.

Mantras, yantras, and mandalas used in tattwa shuddhi have nothing to do with religion, occultism, or mysticism. They should be regarded as highly charged forces who intend to create the same frequency in man that the mantra, yantra, or mandala carries to raise consciousness.

VISUALIZATION AND FANTASY

To create, one must first and foremost be able to visualize and fantasize. Imagination is a mental ability that can be used in all ways. When you make an inner world of visions and symbols, the power of the mind becomes more robust. In tantra, visualization and imagination link the objective and subjective worlds. Tantric visualizations serve as a guide for the practitioner, a medium to concentrate on. In tattwa shuddhi, you want to make the practitioner experience their inner self by creating colors, sounds and images, and visualization of these in concrete form. The pictures are both grotesque and pleasant. The practitioner has clear guidelines to follow to help him reach deeper. In the beginning, you experience the images as thoughts, which, over time, develop into clear, inner images.

THE PERFORMANCE OF PAPA PURUSHA
– the sinful man.

The meditation exercises in tattwa shuddhi consist of many unusual fantasies. The most bizarre of these is Papa Purusha. Papa Purusha symbolizes the cause of suffering, conflict, disharmony and imbalance caused by ego, jealousy, pride, etc. During the exercise, you imagine how Papa Purusha is transformed and takes shape, meaning you change yourself. Papa Purusha's transformation refers to the inner transformation. The transformation and conflict between the negative and positive forces (ida and pingala) constantly strive to unite and transform into the third neutral force. This conflict acts as a catalyst for our evolution and causes us to continue to seek balance in life. In our search for balance, we turn to the spiritual paths, which guide our evolution further and further forward. We would remain complacent and lazy without the conflict between the opposites of energies. Tantra emphasizes the importance of experiencing conflict to create harmony.

The performance of papa purusha is covered on the stage during the exercise when you have become the experience. You witness every action and thought. Each reaction is assessed objectively. Only then, when one can look at oneself objectively, can one see the sides of one's personality that the ego has previously hidden, ages you would rather not see or know about. Here, too, tantra emphasizes the importance of daring to see oneself as one is, not as one wants to be. Only then do you have the opportunity to change yourself.

BHASMA

Tattwa shuddhi is a symbolic act where one lubricates the body with ash (bhasma) to cleanse the body physically and subtly. The great yogi Shiva, the father of tantra, is often depicted sitting naked and anointed in ashes. Lubricating oneself with bhasma favors the experience and discovery of one's own Shiva nature.

Bhasma means "dissolution" or "decomposition" and refers to the decomposition of matter using fire or water. The "bhasmatic" form of matter is produced, which is considered a purer and finer form than the original and all impurities disappear. All matter must finally undergo this process to transform into the fine essential form. It also applies to us humans. To cleanse means the elimination of slag and impurities. The application of bhasma symbolizes our inner conscious-ness's journey from rough matter to pure consciousness.

Bhasma is also used in Ayurveda as a medical treatment method. Bhasma can be made of gold, silver, copper, or other metals. In tattwa shuddhi, cow dung is used. Cow dung is used in India daily as it is considered antibacterial, antiviral, and generally beneficial to the skin. The reason why you use cow dung in tattwa shuddhi and no other substance is essential. By dissolving the cow dung with the help of agni (fire) one reduces it to its bhasmatic form which symbolizes the dis-solution of our senses which we try to do in tattwa shuddhi. Through pratyahara, we loosen up the experience of the objective world and our surroundings. Through dharana, we concentrate the knowledge of what is left to experience, and through dhyana, we broaden this experience to its original cosmic essence, the Shiva consciousness.

In tattwa shuddhi, bhasma is applied to the forehead at the same time as the mantra is pronounced towards the end of the exercise—most people who have done this experience feeling deeply cleansed. Rishis and yogis have used bhasma throughout the ages, and its beneficial effect has led to the technology being used even today.

THE EFFECT OF TATTWA SHUDDHI SADHANA

The effects of tattwa shuddhi are faster and more powerful when compared to other sadhana, as it is a tantric upasana that one dedicates to Shakti, the energy principle behind everything. The effects manifest themselves both materially and as mental forces (siddhis). However, it is essential to remember to perform tattwa shuddhi correctly so as not to create imbalances and obstacles that interfere with the continued spiritual development. It is important to learn the technique from a knowledgeable teacher or guru. Regularity is essential for the exercise, different from how often you practice. We want to train the mind, intellect, and consciousness in tantra. We want to be able to control it with our willpower. It teaches us that regular practice is essential.

PHYSICALLY

The combination of fasting and tattwa shuddhi contributes to changes throughout our physical body. When we cleanse the elements (tattwas) that our body is built of, our heart, liver, kidneys, pancreas and all other organs are affected. Tissues and cells are renewed and given new energy, contributing to a healthier body and mind. Bhasma has a cooling effect on the body and nervous system, which can be heated during intense meditation.

MENTALLY

By visualizing and concentrating on tattwa yantras, chanting mantras, and creating mandalas, we purify samskaras that can be manifested through dreams, visions, and thoughts in our conscious mind. Mental visions are a common effect of most yogic exercises, but within tattwa shuddhi these are usually stronger when one has developed a sharp inner consciousness. You can experience these as subtle sounds, smells, a feeling on the skin, or as taste and shape.

SIDDHIS

Yoga shastras clearly describe that siddhis can be achieved by concentrating on tattwas. By awakening tattwas, one develops higher abilities such as clairvoyance, telepathy, and intuition. The earth's elements help cure diseases and make the body light. Apas tattwa evens the flow of prana in the body and enables astral travel. Agni tattwa can turn base metals into precious metals. Vayu tattwa provides knowledge about the past, present, and future. Akasha tattwa develops mental projection and reveals metaphysical reality. Despite this, siddhis are not what we strive for in tattwa shuddhi; the purpose is higher spiritual experiences that involve the knowledge of the subtle forces that permeate the entire universe. You thus become more receptive to these forces. You naturally become more intuitive and experience bliss on all levels. In tantric texts, one can also read that the knowledge of the elements leads one to freedom from suffering. It is done by knowing that all matter is perishable and that the human body results from atoms, molecules, and energy particles. You stop attaching to things and matter when you know what they consist of – i.e., composite energy.

TATTWA SHUDDHI

PERFORMANCE

*Before you start practicing tattwa shuddhi, you and your teacher /
guru should take a sankalpa regarding how long and often you should
practice. It is said that a sankalpa should be as short as one day. The
person's willpower and mental ability should be considered when de-
termining the period. A sankalpa must always be completed. You can
start practicing at any time during the year, but it is said that July-Au-
gust (Shravan) or October (Ashwin, the month of devi worship) gives
the best results.*

*It would help if you looked after your diet during exercise. Heavy food
makes the body sluggish and slow, is difficult for the body to digest, and
can make it harder to be receptive to higher energies. Salt, solid spices,
and beverages should be avoided as they increase digestion and can
cause too much acid to form. Light foods like dairy products, fruits,
and cooked vegetables are preferred. If you have decided to do tattwa
shuddhi daily, or for some other reason can not keep a light diet, you
should adjust the diet to what is best suited. The special requirements
regarding fasting and diet do not need to be followed if one does not
have a strict sadhana and only practices tattwa shuddhi once a day.*

*According to tradition, tattwa shuddhi should be practiced three times
a day. During Brahma muhurta (before sunrise), afternoon, and
sandhya (dusk). Before the exercise, wash yourself. You should practice
in a quiet, calm place with few impressions and sit facing north or east.
Before the exercise, light a candle and read out your sankalpa. During
the last day, practice mouna, and after the previously completed exercise, sit and meditate on the formless reality.*

Step 1: Preparation.

Practice trataka or pranayama for ten to fifteen minutes before the exercise to calm the mind and go deeper into yourself (pratyahara). Sit in a comfortable meditation position, close your eyes, and practice kaya sthairyam.

Visualize the form of your guru or spiritual guide and feel reverence for them.

Take your attention to the Mooladhara chakra and imagine how the Kundalini Shakti rises upwards with the sushumna nadi to the Sahasrara chakra on top of the head. Meditate on the mantra So Ham, synchronize with breathing: So on inhalation, from Mooladhara to Sahasrara, and Ham on exhalation from Sahasrara to Mooladhara. Experience the movement of the mantra and the breathing as if it were the movement of your inner consciousness.

Step 2: The creation of tattwa yantras.

Take consciousness to the area between the toes and knees. Visualize the shape of a yellow square, the yantra for prithvi tattwa, the earth's element. Experience its golden yellow color and weight. At the same time, repeat the bija mantra, Lam.

Move your attention to the area between the knees and the navel. Visualize a horizontal crescent moon with two white lotus flowers at each end. A circle of water surrounds the crescent. It is the yantra of the apas tattwa, the element of water. Repeat with the mantra Vam.

Move the attention further to the area between the navel and the heart. Visualize a red upside-down triangle burning, the yantra for agni tattwa, the element of fire. Simultaneously repeat the mantra Ram.

Now, focus on the area between the heart and the eyebrow center. Visualize a blue hexagon, which is yantra for the vayu tattwa. Repeat with the mantra Yam.

Move your attention to the area between the eyebrow's center and the head's top. Imagine a circle, the yantra of akasha tattwa, the element of space / ether. In the circle is shoonya (the emptiness), black or filled with multicolored dots. Repeat the mantra, Ham.

Step 3: Resolution of the elements.

Take consciousness back to prithvi yantra. Experience how its form becomes fluid and turns into apas, apas into agni, agni into vayu, and vayu into akasha.

Now imagine how the aksha is transformed into its origin, the aham-kara, the ego.

The ego is then transformed into the mahat tattwa, the great principle. Mahat tattwa dissolves and becomes Prakriti, Prakriti to Purusha (the highest self).

Consider yourself the highest principle, pure and complete.

Step 4: Transformation of the lower nature.

Pay attention to the left side of the abdomen / stomach. Visualize there a tiny man as big as your thumb. He is called Papa Purusha. His skin was black as soot, and he had glowing eyes and a big belly. He holds an ax in one hand and a shield in the other. He is grotesque in form. You will now transform this man with the help of breathing and mantras.

Hold the right nostril with your right thumb and inhale through the left nostril. At the same time, repeat the mantra Yam four times. Visualize how his face and body transform.

Hold both nostrils. Hold your breath and, at the same time, repeat the mantra Ram four times. See how the little man is burned to ashes.

Exhale the ashes through your right nostril while repeating the mantra Vam four times. See how the ashes are rolled into a ball mixed with the moon's nectar in the apas yantra.

Now repeat the mantra, Lam. Imagine how the ball on the left side of your stomach transforms into a golden egg.

Repeat the mantra Ham and simultaneously visualize how the golden egg grows in size and fills your whole body. It feels like you are born again.

Step 5: Re-formation of the elements.

Reshape the elements in reverse order. You again become the highest principle from the golden egg, Prakriti, mahat tattwa, ahamkara.

From ahamkara you see how akasha yantra is created, from akasha

is created vayu, from vayu is created agni, from agni is created apas,
from apas is created prithvi.

Locate the area for each tattwa yantra and repeat the mantra for each
tattwa as before.

Step 6: Kundalini back to Mooladhara.

When you have recreated all the elements, repeat the mantra So Ham
along with the sushumna synchronized with the breathing. Move
the attention from Mooladhara to Sahasrara and from Sahasrara to
Mooladhara.

Experience how you, with the separation of jivatma (your soul), sepa-
rate from paramatma (the cosmic soul). Place jivatma at the heart of
its location.

Visualize the Kundalini Shakti that you directed to the Sahasrara
and experience how it returns down to the Mooladhara through the
sushumna while piercing each chakra on the way down.
Step 7: The shape of the shakti.

Bring your attention to chidakasha. See a giant deep sea in front of you
with a large red lotus flower on the water. On the lotus flower, see the
shape of prana Shakti.

Her body is the same color as a sunrise and decorated with ornaments.
She has three eyes and six arms. In her first hand, she holds a trident;
in the second, a bow made of sugar cane; in the third, a snare; in the
fourth, a spur; in the fifth, five arrows; and the sixth, a skull with blood
dripping from it.

Look at her beautiful shape and say, "May she give us happiness."

Step 8: Application of bhasma.

Become aware of yourself sitting on the floor. Become body conscious. Inhale slowly and deeply. Open your eyes.

Take some bhasma on the middle and ring fingers and slowly pull the fingers on the forehead from left to right while pronouncing the mantra "Om Hraum Namah Shivaya" or "Om Ham Sa" (Sannyasins).

Take bhasma on your thumb, draw a line above the other two lines from right to left, and pronounce the same mantra again.

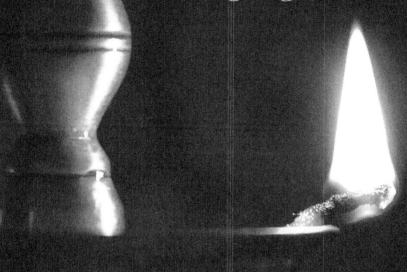

AYURVEDA
The science of Life

AYURVEDA

VATA, PITTA & KAPHA

Ayurveda is an Indian health science with roots in the Vedic tradition. Both yoga and Ayurveda originally came into being as Vedic teachings and are believed to be more than five thousand years old.

Ayur means life, and Veda means knowledge – the knowledge / science about life. With the help of Ayurveda, we can learn to live in balance with our life force and our entire divine consciousness.

In Ayurveda, the whole person is treated, not just the sick. When you create balance, you simultaneously release the self-healing forces. Ayurveda develops the health potential we have within us and, at the same time, expands our consciousness.

Ayurveda and yoga originate from the same tradition and have been practiced together for thousands of years. It is often forgotten, resulting in yoga and Ayurveda being taught separately. Both classical yoga and Ayurveda take the whole person into account physically, mentally, and spiritually.

You could say that Ayurveda is a tradition of Vedic knowledge that describes how to heal the body and mind, while yoga is a tradition of Vedic knowledge that describes the path to self-insight. Achieving self-insight requires that the body and mind are in balance.

UPAVEDAS

Ayurveda is part of the four upavedas that supplement the four Vedas.

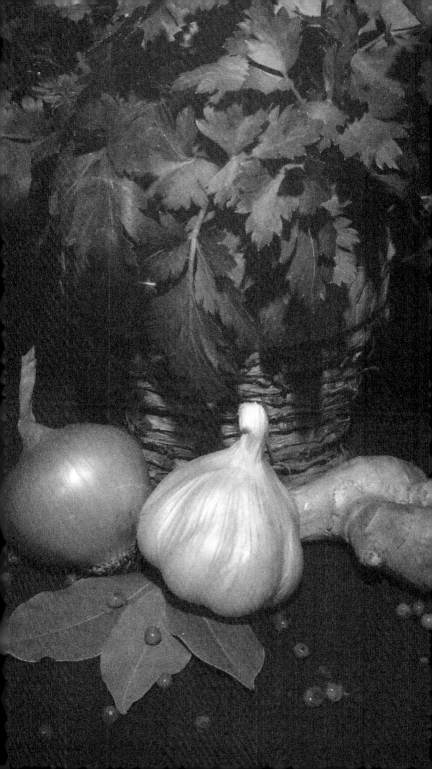

Ayurveda is also closely related to the practice of Veda as it treats various mantras and methods to cure diseases. The four upavedas are:

1. Ayurveda – knowledge of life.

2. Gandharva veda – knowledge of culture, art and music's role in spiritual development. For example, there is music for various disease conditions.

3. Dhanur veda – knowledge of the importance of behavior for spiritual development.

4. Sthapatya veda – knowledge of the importance of architecture for spiritual development. This veda is also known as vastu and is reminiscent of feng shui. Feng Shui is a philosophy that practices arranging building structures and objects within living spaces to create balance and energy.

THREE DOSHAS

In Ayurveda, three doshas or energy principles control all life processes internally and externally. Our biological existence is based on the interplay between these three energy principles. Doshas combines the five elements: space, air, fire, water, and earth.

The doshas also determine what personality type you are. It is usually said that you have one or two doshas that dominate. According to astrology, the influence of the celestial bodies (grahas) during conception determines which dosha becomes the most dominant in each person. There is dosha type one, dosha type two, and dosha type three.

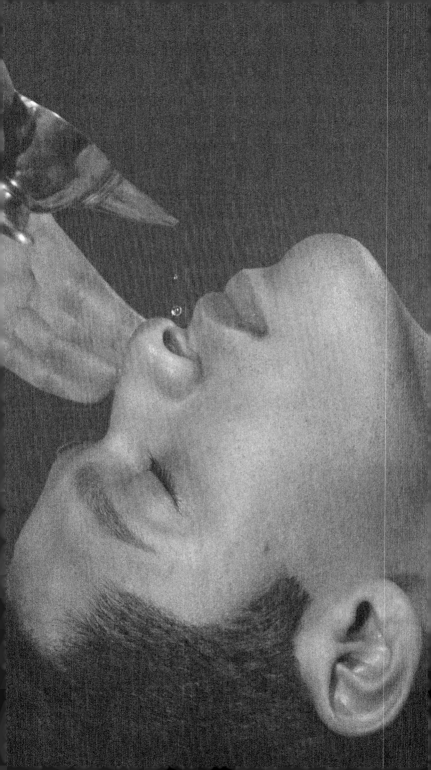

In our yoga practice, it is essential to understand how the doshas affect us. Knowing the energy principles and how they act and interact in and around us, we can take full advantage of fine yogic techniques to create balance and harmony in our physical and subtle bodies. We can adapt our yoga practice to the needs and personality types that we need to achieve the best possible results.

In Ayurveda, yoga is used to maintain a healthy lifestyle and as a treatment method for diseases. Asanas, pranayamas, and meditation are among the best methods to maintain balance in the doshas.

VATA	PITTA	KAPHA
Space / air.	*Fire / water.*	*Water / soil.*
Movement.	*Combustion.*	*Structure.*
Dry.	*A little oily.*	*Fat / oily.*
Light.	*Light.*	*Heavy.*
Cold.	*Warm / hot.*	*Cold.*
Very fast.	*Fast.*	*Slow.*
Hearing / feeling.	*The eyes.*	*Taste / smell.*
The moon.	*The sun.*	*Earth.*

Vata is kinetic energy in various ways and the force that allows the other two doshas to move. Vata exists as air in our organs, joints, and bones. On a deeper level, vata is the life force within us and the power of thought that moves in our minds. Vata controls the central nervous system, the movements of the heart, the intestines, the lungs, the thought processes, and the communication between the mind and the body.

Pitta is responsible for the metabolism and conversion process in the body. In addition to digestion, it melts our impressions of the outside world, emotions, and ideas. Pitta provides us with intelligence, courage, and vitality. With pitta, we gain motivation and sight to reach our goals in life. You can see pitta in photosynthesis, which is nature's combustion.

Kapha is the one who unites. The stable structure is associated with bone structure, mucous membranes, joints, rocks, and mountains. Kapha provides us with emotions and feelings that contribute to love, care, devotion, and faith, which causes us to maintain harmony within ourselves and unite with others.

Vata, pitta, and kapha are closely linked and always work together. In every single cell in the body, these three interact. For vata to be in balance, pitta and kapha must exist in the right proportion because they have these elements in the form of water and fire. Vata is the easiest to get out of balance but also the easiest to rebalance. Pitta, in turn, needs to be watered with vata's properties of movement and decomposition (start the fire / dampen the fire) and also kapha's building and preserving properties to keep the fire alive. Kapha needs vata to start the movement and pitta for its stimulus and warming properties. Conse-

quently, we see that none of the doshas can exist without the other; they are all equally important.

RAJAS, TAMAS & SATTVA

Prakriti consists of three varying qualities: rajas, tamas, and sattva. Rajas is the active, stimulating, and positive force contributing to change. Tamas is the passive and harmful force that keeps the old. Sattva is the neutral and balancing force that harmonizes the positive and the negative. All three energies are necessary for everything that happens, even on the spiritual plane.

Sattva is the light, the love, and the life. It is the higher spiritual power that makes us develop our consciousness. Rajas is the passion, the twilight, and what changes. It is the vital force that lacks stability. It gives rise to emotional fluctuations such as fear and desire, love and hate. Tamas is the dark, the insensitive, and the dead. The lower material force pulls us to unconsciousness, stagnation, listlessness, and heaviness. Unmanifested Prakriti keeps these three in balance. Rajas and tamas get sattva together. When Prakriti is manifested, these qualities are distinguished.

Sattva gives rise to the mind, rajas generates the life force, and tamas stands for form and substance as the physical body. Yoga and Ayurveda want to develop the sattvic state. In yoga, sattva is the higher quality that makes us grow spiritually. In Ayurveda, sattva is the state of balance in which the healing property is released.

YOGIC AND AYURVEDIC DIET

In Ayurveda, diet plays a considerable role and lays the foundation for all other therapeutic approaches and healing processes. Without a pro-

per and balanced diet, other medicines have no significant effect. The food is used as medicine. A sattvic diet is advocated because sattva creates balance. A sattvic diet is traditionally based on ahimsa, an ethical principle of not causing harm to other living beings. As far as possible, the food should have grown naturally in a harmonious environment as such food carries a lot of prana and pure awareness.

Yogis worldwide are usually very aware of what they eat, but a traditional yogic diet and an Ayurvedic one are different. Ayurveda wants to create balance and build good physical health. In yoga, you want to develop and change body awareness. In short, Ayurveda wants to make physical health, and yoga helps us get beyond the body's limits. Many traditional yogic paths are ascetic, where solid, simple raw foods with detoxifying effects are common. However, these have a water-raising impact. A Standard Ayurvedic diet is instead based on well-cooked and nutritious food to strengthen us physically and prevent doshas from becoming unbalanced or unnecessarily wet.

A traditional yogic diet increases the elements of space / ether and air (vata) to detoxify and open up the mind. Therefore, raw food and fasting are recommended. By reducing the body, you expand the mind. Another significant factor in the yogic diet is prana. A raw diet is rich in prana. By following a raw diet, you increase the flow of prana in the body and thus purify nadis. Breathing exercises improve the digestive fire in the body, allowing the food to be digested even though it's not cooked.

However, only some of us can digest this type of food satisfactorily. It is especially true for vata people with varying digestive fire, but even kapha and pitta can have difficulty with this. Therefore, most non-ascetics feel better from a well-cooked, warm diet that is easy to digest.

An Ayurvedic diet is not necessarily sattvic but focuses more on creating physical health. On the other hand, a Yogic diet places the most significant emphasis on the food's satiety, which can increase a dosha. You can choose sattvic food adapted to your dominant dosha type for an optimal diet. Sattvic food includes dairy products, natural oils, herbal teas, sweet spices, fruits, fresh juices, vegetables, cereals, legumes, nuts, seeds, and honey. For a sattvic diet, eating the correct type of food at the right time during the day is divided into vata, pitta, and kapha time. In Ayurveda, it is recommended to eat light food for breakfast because Kapha time prevails, and heavy food also weighs down the mind and body. The biggest goal should be to eat in the middle of the day during pitta time when digestion is at its strongest. In the evening, you should not eat heavy foods or too close to bedtime as it disturbs both sleep and the natural cleansing of waste materials.

THE SIX TASTES
Six different flavors affect each dosha in different ways. Each flavor consists of a combination of two elements.

Sweet – water and soil.
Balances vata and pitta. It increases kapha—for example, vegetables, oils, milk and rice.

Sour – fire and soil.
Balances vata. It increases pitta and kapha—for example, citrus, yogurt, cheese, and vinegar.

Salt – fire and water.
Balances vata. It increases pitta and kapha—for example, seaweed, tamari, and table salt.

Pungent – fire and air.
It decreases kapha. It increases pitta and vata—for example, strong spices such as pepper, onion, and ginger.

Bitter – space and air.
Balances pitta and kapha. It increases vata—for example, green leafy vegetables and turmeric.

Astringent – air and soil.
Balances pitta and kapha. It increases vata—for example, beans, lentils, and unripe bananas.

TIP
Try to eat in silence and in a relaxed manner. Focus on the meal and not on anything else at the same time. Eat foods you like and avoid cold foods. Avoid eating when you feel anxious, angry, or sad. Drink boiled water with food, not milk. Eat freshly prepared food as much as possible and avoid leftovers, as the nutrients have already been lost. The food must be equipped with love and awareness.

AGNI
In Ayurveda, the body's digestive fire – agni, is significant. If the fire is too weak, the food cannot be digested satisfactorily, and nutrients are lost. The food we eat then becomes ama (slag products), which strains our bodies. In Ayurveda, a weak digestive fire is the root cause of most diseases. Our modern life and our stress are major contributing factors to poor digestion. We tend to gulp down food instead of enjoying it.

When we have a balance between the doshas, the agni will also be in balance. A sign of this is when we regularly feel a healthy appetite.

The agni is weakened when we overeat, snack, or eat even though we are not hungry. Refrigerated food, prolonged fasting, and poorly chewed food are also contributing factors.

When vata is increased, digestion becomes irregular. It can change from fast to slow; sometimes, you can feel an intense hunger. Stomach problems are also part of the picture.

When pitta gets out of balance, the agni becomes too strong. You may experience extreme hunger, often shortly after eating. It contributes to nutrients not being absorbed by the body, and in the long run, you can suffer from stomach ulcers.

When kapha is elevated, digestion becomes very slow instead. You experience a heavy feeling after eating, and feelings of hunger are weak.

AGNI YOGA

Both yoga and Ayurveda carry the knowledge of the divine fire, the agni. We learn to control the fire to create balance and to develop. The cosmic fire exists everywhere, in ourselves and around us. In the body, we see the agni in the form of our digestive fire; on a finer level, the agni corresponds to our eternal consciousness. Without fire, our development and evolution will stop.

In Ayurveda, we learn to balance the function of the agni physically by taking care of our digestive fire, which then lays the foundation for good health.

In yoga, the focus is on the pranic agni and the fire of meditation, which are essential for our enlightenment. Various fire rituals are performed every day in yoga traditions. Still, we may be most familiar with the Breath of Fire exercise, which cleanses the body's energy channels and increases the flow of prana in the body.

YOGA'S IMPACT ON OUR THREE DOSHAS

ASANAS AND AYURVEDA

Asanas release tension and energy blockages that may have occurred, thereby keeping the body's tissues, joints, and organs in the best possible shape. The positions stretch and strengthen the muscles, and the spine is kept flexible, making it possible for the energy to flow freely through nerves that belong to our organs and glands. Our tissues are, therefore, cleansed systematically, preparing the body for more advanced yogic exercises.

Asanas prepare you for breathing exercises and meditation. They not only have a physical purpose, but they also affect us on a practical, mental, and spiritual level. From the beginning, asanas have aimed to counter rajas, the turbulent energy within us that distracts the mind.

Asanas help to balance and release the prana in the body, which pre-pares us for breathing exercises. Our senses are turned inward, which facilitates mind control (pratyahara). When our thoughts are still, the mind is calmed so that we can concentrate (dharana) and meditate (dhyana).

Diet and asanas are the two most essential factors in creating good health and counteracting imbalances and diseases in the long run.

Spices, herbs, and various breathing exercises are used to balance the prana in the body. A proper posture and diet are required as a basis to enable this. Our posture is of great importance for our health and cons

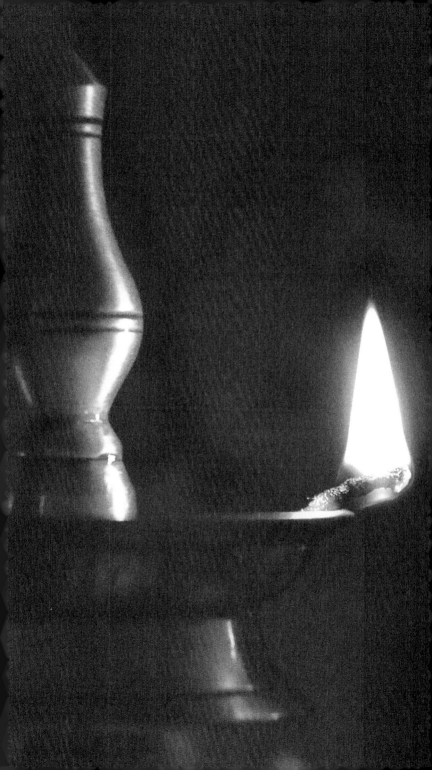

ciousness. The body and the mind influence each other through subtle channels in the body through which foods and our thoughts flow. The musculoskeletal system holds the channels together, the shape of which is determined by our posture. Improper posture causes stress in the body and blocks these channels. The energy cannot flow optimally, and residual products and toxins have a chance to accumulate. It eventually leads to discomfort in the body, pain, and illness.

It is easy for asanas to become the mainstay of yoga practice. If you want to participate in yoga on a deeper level, give equal time to asanas, pranayamas, and meditation. An exaggerated and unconscious execution of asanas leads to a fixation on the body and boosts our physical ego: this leads to a rigid and undeveloped mind and emotions. Never exaggerate the exercises or force the body into a position that will cause more tension and injury.

ASANAS AND OUR AGE

Infants and children are by nature soft and flexible in the body. Practicing asanas early means maintaining the softness and correct posture for life.

Vinyasas are suitable for younger people because many rajas prevail in body and mind, and they need vinyasas to mature. After twenty-four, one should move on to inner yoga and develop the mind by studying yogic texts.

After forty-eight, the mind develops at the same speed as the physical energies are withdrawn. It would help if you meditate more, but asanas are still crucial for keeping the body supple and healthy.

At sixty–five, the vata age, the body fluids slowly decrease and dry out. The body becomes stiffer, and joint diseases are common. With the help of asanas, you can keep your body in shape and balance excess vata.

At the age of seventy-two, the mind develops even more. It is the time for deep meditation. Asanas continue to be essential to slow down aging.

ASANAS FOR VATA

Vata people often have a slim and thin physique. They are very flexible and mobile when young but quickly develop stiffness as they age. Vatas often suffer from joint problems in middle age. They are often cold, have dry skin, cracked joints, and poor blood circulation. Vata people are naturally nervous and scared, which makes them tense in their shoulders and back. Asanas are essential for vata people, for both their health and their ability to meditate. Vatas must exercise caution when practicing asanas as they are prone to injury. Soft, flowing exercises at a reasonable speed are preferred.

Mental preparation is essential for vatas: a moment of rest and deep breathing before asanas is necessary. During practice, vatas should start slowly so the circulation awakens and the joints can warm up. Vatas should not be too sweaty as they dry out quickly. Intake of fluid is essential. Asanas should mainly affect the area around the hips and intestines, which is the main seat of vata. Releasing tension from the hips and lumbar spine is essential. Too much stretching and movement can cause over-stretching and weakness.

Sitting positions such as padmasana and vajrasana are good for vata. These have a calming, grounding effect and control apana vayu.

Keeping the spine flexible is essential for vatas, who often accumulate tension here. Exercises that rotate the spine in each direction are good. Matsyendrasana is an example of a pose that releases vata from the nervous system. It is essential to have proper breathing when performing spinal rotation. Otherwise, the pose will have the opposite effect and increase vata.

Forward bending positions have a calming effect and release vata from the back. Combining forward-turning positions with backward-bending positions is essential to maximize the benefits. However, this should be done slowly and carefully. Doing backward bending positions too quickly can stimulate the sympathetic nervous system and our "fight or flight" mechanism. With caution, asanas such as the cobra and the grasshopper have a grounding and strengthening effect on vatas.

Standing poses are perfect for vata. They build strength, give peace, and increase stability.

Vatas should avoid becoming too exhausted. Dynamic asanas should be accompanied by sitting positions, pranayamas, and meditation.

After asanas, vatas should lie and rest in shavasana. It is an optimal time to meditate, with the mind calm and the emotions stable.

Seated poses:
Siddhasana / siddha yoni asana (perfect pose), vajrasana (diamond pose) and simhasana (lion pose).

The sun salutation:
Slowly and consciously.

Standing poses:
Vrksasana (tree pose), trikonasana (triangle pose), virabhadrasana (warrior pose), parighasana (gate pose), and all standing forward bending positions.

Inverted poses:
Shirshasana (headstand), vipareeta karani asana (half shoulder stand).

Backbends:
Bhujangasana (cobra) and shalabhasana (grasshopper).

Forward bends:
All. Especially janu sirsasana (half-butterfly) and pachimottasana (pliers).

Spinal twists:
Lying positions, bharadvajasana (half turn) and shava udarakarshanasana (universal position).

Other:
Shashankasana (hare), parivrtta janu sirsasana (one-legged forward bend in a seated position), navasana (boat), yoga mudra.

Shavasana:
At least twenty minutes.

ASANAS FOR PITTA

Pittas have a medium-sized physique. They often have good muscles and flexibility. Circulation and joint mobility are usually good due to the slightly oily nature of pittas. Pittas usually handle asanas very well, but if overdone, it may lead to hypermobility and stiffness in joints.

Mentally, pitta people are aggressive and like to shine in everything they do. Pittas must be careful about "performing" when it comes to asanas. They can often become perfect at technical but need to remember the spiritual part. Pittas often need to be more ambitious, annoyed, and very driven. Asanas should be used to cool pittas down physically and mentally, helping them turn their intelligence inward to understand themselves better.

Calm breathing and sitting still after powerful asanas are essential to counteract stress. Pittas should avoid overly strenuous exercise and not get too hot. Powerful asanas are ok as long as pittas compensate by using cooling asanas and pranayamas to cool the mind and body towards the end.

Around the navel, heat is created and distributed throughout the body. We have a cooling function in the palate, where saliva is secreted. The heat from the umbilical region moves upwards to reduce the cold produced in the soft palate. The cooling property is protected from heat by standing in a shoulder position or entering the plow position. These positions reverse the positions of the sun and the moon in the body, which creates balance, especially in pitta people. Spinal twists such as matsyendrasana are also suitable for protecting the cooling property without lowering the fire in the body. Positions that release tension and affect the abdominal tract, small intestine, and liver are also beneficial for pittas because pittas accumulate in these areas. The bow, cobra, boat, and fish poses are good. Headstand increases pitta and should be avoided if you do not know how to balance the heat afterward.

Forward bending positions are generally suitable for pittas because they increase the energy around the abdomen and have a cooling and grounding effect. Back-bending positions create more heat and should, therefore, be practiced in moderation and followed by cooling asanas. Seated spinal twists help cleanse the liver and detoxify the pitta.

After asanas, pitta should feel calm, cool, and relaxed in the stomach. The mind should be in a meditative state and not too sharp.

Seated poses:
Most are beneficial except simhasana (the lion), which should be avoided.

The moon greeting:
Cooling for pitta.

Standing poses:
Vrksasana (tree pose), trikonasana (triangle pose), ardha chandrasana (crescent pose).

Standing poses (legs wide apart):
Moordhasana (head on the floor from standing with legs apart), pa-dottanasana (leg lift).

Forward bends:
All seated forward bends are good, especially pada prasar paschi-

mottanasana (forward bend with legs split), kurmasana (turtle) and paschimottanasana (pliers).

Twists:
Ardha matsyendrasana (half spinal rotation).

Other:
Sarvangasana (shoulder stand), vipareeta karani (half shoulder stand), navasana (boat), ardha matsyendrasana (seated spine twisting), bhu-jangasana (cobra), yoga mudra.

Shavasana:
Medium, long.

ASANAS FOR KAPHA

Kapha types are heavily built and gain weight quickly. They are often inflexible and should not try to push the body into a position like a lotus position, which carries a risk of injury. Kapha's body and joints often do not support these positions. Kaphas must accept how they are built and not try to become thin, slim yogis because their body is not made that way.

Kapha women can be thin when young but gain weight over the years, especially after giving birth. It can weigh down kaphas as they may have difficulty accepting this. In this case, they are expected to use different ways to try to lose weight, such as yoga, although it rarely results. Kaphas must instead work on their attitude toward their body and accept what is natural for them. Kaphas still needs to try to maintain average body weight without starving themselves.

Obesity in kapha is mainly seen on the abdomen and thighs, causing various problems with posture. Increased kapha also causes mucus formation around the breasts and lungs, spreading to different parts of the body and causes duct blockages. These blockages contribute to increased fat accumulation around joints and tissues.

Kapha people are rarely physically active, although needing it to stimulate their metabolism and increase circulation. As kaphas are easily affected by high cholesterol and heart disease, they should exercise cautiously and be mindful not to overwork while still challenging themselves.

As heat triggers the flow in kaphas, exercises that increase heat and make the body sweat are good. Kaphas needs to be pushed to do strenuous exercises that they do not think they can do.

Sitting asanas increase kapha. Pranayamas that increase heat are beneficial before meditation.

Vinyasas such as the sun salutation are good to start the flow. Backward bending positions are also good as they open up the chest, which is the area for kapha. Backbends also increase circulation in the head, which counteracts inertia. Forward bending positions should generally be avoided by kaphas unless they need to calm the nervous system.

Kaphas often suffer from slow digestion. Therefore, exercises like the arch that initiates the flow at the navel region are excellent. The plow is one of the best positions to open up the lungs. Pranayamas create the flow in both body and mind.

After asanas, kaphas should feel light and warm and have increased circulation in the body. The chest and lungs should be open, and the mind should feel clear and alert.

Seated poses:
Simhasana (the lion) and in combination with pranayamas.

The sun salutation:
At a fast pace.

Standing poses:
Virabhadrasana (warrior), Utthita hasta padangusthasana (hand-to-toe stand), bakasana (crow), ardha chandrasana (crescent position).

Inverted poses:
Adho mukha vrksasana (downward facing dog), sirsasana (headstand), sarvangasana (shoulder stand).

Backbends:
Ustrasana (camel pose), shalabasana (grasshopper pose).

Other:
Shava udarakarshanasana (spinal rotation), ardha matsyendrasana (half spinal rotation), parvatasana (mountain pose), and halasana (plow pose).

Shavasana:
Short.

PRANAYAMAS

Yoga teaches us how to master prana and thus gain access to its more profound powers. When we learn that, we no longer need external pleasure. In this way, we take control of our mind and can heal it and our body. A knowledgeable Ayurveda doctor knows how to redirect the prana in the body to heal the patient. In the same way, food, herbs, and other healing methods influence the prana.

Pranayama is one of the most central exercises in yoga and is the fourth step in classical yoga. The prana cleanses and revitalizes the body before meditation.

With breathing exercises, you slow down and prolong your breath. It causes the life energy – the prana, to manifest itself.

Breathing exercises have a good effect on diseases that affect the respiratory organs, circulation, and nervous system, as well as fatigue and a weak immune system. The whole body is affected by the exercises by massaging the internal organs. The circulation increases in the internal organs and is detoxified. Pranayamas also have an excellent effect on depression, stress, and tension.

PRANA AND APANA

The apana associated with gravity moves downwards and results in disease, aging, death, and unconsciousness. Prana, related to the elements of air and space, moves upwards through our senses. Combining these two energies can strengthen our energy and awaken our higher abilities. Yogic exercises involve redirecting the apana upwards to meet the prana and pulling the prana down to meet the apana. It takes place at the solar plexus, which is the seat of the prana.

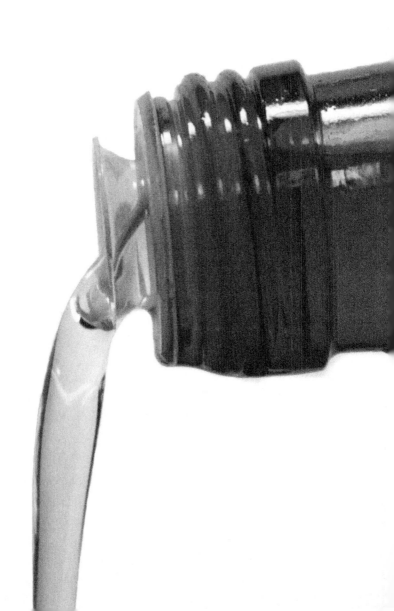

Prana – inhalation.

Samana – hold your breath / contract.

Vyana – hold your breath / expand.

Udana – exhale / squeeze out.

Apana – exhale / elimination.

PRANAYAMA AND PRANA AGNI

Pranayamas develop the fire of prana, which is responsible for the body's combustion. It is done by holding your breath. Oxygen acts as food for pranaagni. The carbon dioxide that accompanies the exhalation is its residual product. Holding our breath cleanses our subtle body in the same way that fasting cleanses our physical. Prana agni gives power to Kundalini so it can continue its journey upwards and take with it prana and apana.

PRANAYAMAS AND DOSHAS

Pranayamas affect all doshas. Done correctly, they help balance vata, reduce kapha, and counter pitta. Inhalation relates to kapha and has a constructive effect. Holding the breath in links to the pitta and is having a transforming impact. Exhalation relates to vata and has a reducing effect.

Breathing through the right nostril gives power to the pingala nadi and increases pitta. Breathing through the left nostril gives power to ida nadi and increases kapha. Balanced breathing through both nostrils balances vata.

Kapha increases when you breathe through your mouth, which is generally advised against. However, there are some specific breathing exercises where you apply breathing through the mouth which can help the prana to be retained in the sushumna nadi.

VATA

Breathing through the right nostril is revitalizing for vata. Practice with intent in the morning for about ten to fifteen minutes. Breathing through the left nostril has a calming effect and calms the mind. Practice with purpose in the evening to improve night sleep. Bhastrika can help energize and clarify the mind, but it should be done carefully. End the exercise if dizziness occurs.

PITTA

Cooling pranayamas are best suited for pittas. Breathing through the left nostril is beneficial in the evening and in cases of feeling overheated or irritated. Shitali and sitkari pranayamas have an excellent effect on strong overheating, irritation and emotions.

KAPHA

Breathing through the right nostril is well suited for the morning as it reduces kapha. Bhastrika and kapalbhati are excellent for kaphas, especially for countering the effects of colds (not fever), listlessness and depression.

MEDITATION

Meditation consists mainly of dharana (concentration), dhyana (meditation), and samadhi (ecstasy). These three steps belong to the inner aspect of the eight steps of yoga. In Ayurveda, meditation is used for therapeutic purposes, mainly to heal the mind and psychological diseases. Still, its effect also affects our physical body as our physical body is also affected by our mental state. The body, prana, and senses must be balanced to meditate.

Both the body and the mind are made up of the five elements. The body comprises elements heavy in character, such as earth and water (kapha), which shape our body. The body's functions consist of slightly lighter elements and doshas. Pitta (fire) is responsible for bodily transformations, while vata (air) is responsible for the impulses between our brain and nerve impulses. The mind is made up of the lighter form of vata (air and ether), which makes it volatile. The mind's functions consist of the heavier elements: fire, water, and earth (pitta and kapha). Fire gives the mind perceptions, the water adds emotions, and the earth connects the mind with the body. The mind is fast and in perpetual change.

Vatas are more quick-witted than other dosha types. It is easier for them to make new acquaintances (air) and be open to new experiences (ether). Vatas have very active senses and are always on the move somewhere. They are more often affected by mental and psychological imbalances.

Pitta is seen as the insightful part of the mind, with the third eye of the mind relating to the element of fire. The fire of reason is called buddhi (intellect and insight). Pitta types are often brilliant, with an excellent ability to focus and have sharp and clear thinking.

Kaphas feel emotions, love, and devotion linked to our senses and the external character of the mind (manas). Bliss, as the core of the mind, is the highest form of kapha.

Meditation allows us to come in contact with our higher self and consciousness (atman and purusha). With the help of meditation, we can cleanse our subconscious from things that cause us suffering. Re-

gardless of the meditation technique used, the purpose is to create the original stillness of our consciousness, which is our true nature.

Meditation can help with:

– Psychological diseases.
– Difficulty falling asleep.
– Emotional disorders.
– Chronic diseases such as allergies and asthma that are affected by stress and hypersensitivity in the nervous system.
– Heart disease. According to ancient Vedic texts, our consciousness belongs to the heart. Therefore, calming the mind and strengthening the heart go hand in hand.
– Pain relief by, e.g., focusing on a mantra.
– Preparing for death and leaving the body.

MEDITATION FOR VATA

Meditation can help vatas with their hypersensitive and active mind to provide better sleep, improve metabolism, and strengthen the immune system. Caution must be exercised as meditation performed incorrectly can have the opposite effect on vatas and cause feelings of volatility. Vatas should first and foremost exercise their ability to concentrate. Techniques that include mantras and visualization are good because they saturate the mind instead of "emptying" it. Vatas should not try to calm the natural flow of thoughts but observe and let it flow.

Preparation:
– Relaxing asanas help vata types sit for more extended periods.
– Deep breathing exercises increase concentration by providing the body with prana.

Visualizations:
– Earth, fire, and water.
– Mountains, lakes, flowers, fire, and sunset.

Balancing colors:
– Gold and saffron help vata types achieve mental clarity.

Mantras:
– Ram, Shrim, and Hrim.
During meditation or when vata seems to be out of balance.

Deities to meditate on:
– Durga and Tara give a feeling of security.
– Shiva and Vishnu give a feeling of security.
– Ganesha creates a sense of grounding.

Considering vata's anxious and fearful nature, devotion to a god or any teacher or guru is suitable. In this way, vatas can leave their worries and problems to someone else, get help, and experience security at the same time.

Vatas must learn to experience contact with the eternal within itself, create stability, and not worry about the changing world. Vatas need space and peace to escape the pace of their surroundings. Meditation on the true eternal helps to slow down one's thoughts.

MEDITATION FOR PITTA
Pitta people need meditation to release emotions such as aggression and anger. They often have an excellent ability to concentrate, and it is easy for them to meditate. Mantra meditation is a perfect way for

pittas to maximize their solid mental energy by focusing it on a goal. Pitta types must work to expand their mind and heart with the help of the inner light and thus gain insight into the truth. The meditation should provide stillness in the mind and heart of the pitta.

Preparation:
– Soothing asanas that do not create too much heat in the body.
– Shitali pranayama, or breathing through the left nostril to cool the system.

Visualizations:
– Mountains, forests, lakes, and seas.
– Rain clouds, flowers in cold colors, the moon and the stars.

Balancing colors:
– White, dark blue, and green.

Affirmations:
– Devotion, love, and forgiveness to balance the fire.
– Prayers for peace and love for other people.

Mantras:
– Shrim, Sham, and Om. Recited silently.

Deities to meditate on:
– Lakshmi, Uma Parvati, Shiva, and Vishnu.

Pittas can be very critical and judgmental. They can use and transform this power by redirecting it to explore their inner self and expand their consciousness. Meditating on infinite space beyond all limitations is beneficial to their critical minds.

MEDITATION FOR KAPHA

Kaphas need meditation to free themselves from old emotional and mental patterns and to counteract inertia. Kaphas need a lot of encouragement and motivation to meditate, so group meditation is usually best suited for them.

It is easy for kaphas to fall asleep and daydream, so choosing an active form of meditation can help prevent this from happening. A combined form of meditation and activity with mantras or pranayamas is good.

Preparation:
– Powerful asanas that start the circulation in the body.
– Bhastrika pranayama, or breathing through the right nostril.

Visualization:
– Fire, air, and ether.
– Sun, wind, sky.

Balancing colors:
– Gold, blue, and orange.

Affirmations:
– Which strengthens the connection to the higher self.
For example. "In my true self, I am independent and free, in nature and space."

Mantras:
– Om, Hum and Aim.
Cleansing and stimulating, to be recited out loud.

Deities to meditate on:
– Shiva and Kali. Divinities of an angry nature release emotions and reduce the ego.

Meditating on emptiness and the inner light creates more space and fire in the mind, which benefits kaphas.

PULSE DIAGNOSTICS

In Ayurveda, various techniques are used to establish a diagnosis of one's health. These include analysis of heart rate, urine, feces, eyes, tongue, speech, skin, shape, and most importantly, pulse. Taking one's pulse as a diagnostic tool has been used in Ayurveda since immemorial. A well-experienced Ayurvedic physicist can use the pulse to assess prakruti (one's general constitution), vikruti (current imbalances in the doshas), subtle imbalances, and other diseases.

You can read the pulse in different places in the body – e.g., in the armpit, ankle, and wrist, of which the latter is the most common. It is done by placing the index finger, middle finger, and ring finger on the upper side of the wrist (towards the thumb). The three fingers represent the different doshas: vata, pitta, and kapha. The index finger represents the vata dosha, the middle finger represents the pitta dosha, and the ring finger represents the kapha dosha. Each dosha has a characteristic pulse: from where the pulse starts, where on the finger it beats the strongest, from which direction it hits, and what quality the pulse has. Rishis use animal movement patterns to describe heart rate levels:

The vata pulse's movement pattern can be compared to how a cobra moves. It is fast, weak, cold, thin, disappears with pressure, and is best felt under the index finger.

The pitta pulse's movement pattern can be compared to a frog. It is prominent, robust, warm, and influential, lifts the palpating finger, and best feels under the middle finger.

The kapha pulse's movement can be likened to a swimming swan. It is deep, slow, wide, wavy, dense, cold or hot, regular, and can be best felt under the ring finger.

THE SEVEN LEVELS OF THE PULSE
In Ayurveda, the pulse is divided into seven levels, each of which tells us how we feel mentally, physically, and spiritually. You can read the different levels by placing three palpating fingers on the wrist and changing the pressure. The pulses provide the practitioner with vikruti (imbalances) in our doshas. Manas vikruti (manas: mind).

SUBDOSHA
Each dosha (vata, pitta, and kapha) has five subdoshas. Each subdosha represents a particular aspect of our physiology. In each subdosha, one of the five elements is prominent.

Vata subdoshas: prana, udana, samana, vyana and apana.

Pitta subdoshas: pachaka, ranjaka, alochaka, sadhaka and bharajaka.

Kapha subdoshas: kledaka, avalambaka, bodhaka, tarpaka and shleshaka.

Prana, tejas and ojas. Prana is the essence of vata, tejas is the essence of pitta, and ojas is the essence of kapha. Ojas are created during nutrition and are the main essence of all tissues. Tejas can be compared to hormones and amino acids. Prana, which is the vital life energy, is responsible for the cooperation between cells.

Dhatus represents our biological tissues, such as plasma, blood, muscle, fat, bones, nerves, and male and female reproductive tissues.

Prakruti represents our basic psychosomatic and biological constitution. Manas Prakruti (manas: sun). If a person says they are, for example, a pitta person, they are not talking about any imbalance but their essential constitution.

CHINESE MEDICINE

Pulse diagnostics is also an essential part of Chinese medicine. However, Ayurvedic pulse diagnostics and Chinese differ somewhat. In Chinese technology, one can read forty-seven aspects of the pulse, compared with the seven levels in Ayurveda.

AYURVEDIC TREATMENTS

In Ayurvedic treatment, there are eight main disciplines, so-called ashtangas:

Internal medicine (kaya-chikitsa).
Pediatrics (kaumarabhrityam).
Surgery (shalya-chikitsa).
Eyes (shalakya-tantra).
The science of demonic obsession (bhuta-vidya). It has been called psychiatry.
Toxicology (agada-tantram).
Disease prevention, immunity enhancement, and rejuvenation (rasayana).
Aphrodisiacs and improving the health of the offspring (vajikaranam).

AYURVEDIC MASSAGE

Ayurvedic massage is used to treat various diseases and for preventive purposes.

There are at least forty different types of Ayurvedic massage, which, along with various other diagnostic tools, are used by Ayurvedic doctors to treat diseases and ill health.

Ayurvedic massage relieves pain, relaxes stiff muscles, reduces swelling caused by joint inflammation, improves blood circulation, increases stress resistance, provides better sleep, increases athletic performance, and provides emotional benefits. With Ayurvedic massage, deeply rooted toxins are released in joints and tissues and eliminated through natural processes.

ABHYANGA – AYURVEDIC OIL MASSAGE

Abhyanga (oil massage) is a standard Ayurvedic massage. Abhyanga is a therapeutic massage of about forty-five minutes and is used to treat many diseases. Two therapists working on the client's side often give Abhyanga, lying on a wooden bed. Particular attention is paid to the feet because there are marma points (nerve nodes) on the soles of the feet that are closely related to specific internal organs. The sole of the right foot is massaged clockwise, and the left is counterclockwise.

During treatment, the client rests in seven standard positions. Abhyanga begins with the client sitting in an upright position, after which she lies flat on her back, turns to the right side, lies on her back again, turns to the left side, lies on her back again, and finally returns to a sitting position. Abhyanga is an essential part of pancha karma therapy.

SHIRO ABHYANGA – AYURVEDIC HEAD MASSAGE

Shiro abhyanga is a head massage with roots in Ayurveda. The purpose of Shiro abhyanga is not only to ward off stress but also to stimulate the body to heal itself. Various oils are usually included as a natural part of the treatment to soothe the soul and care for the skin and hair. Shiro abhyanga is a head massage that, in addition to Ayurvedic contexts, is common in hair salons in India.

NASYAM – AYURVEDIC NASAL TREATMENT

Nasyam is an Ayurvedic treatment in which medicinal oils are administered through the nose to clear the throat, nose, and head of harmful substances.

This treatment is used to treat migraines, headaches, mental disorders, prematurely graying hair, and speech difficulties. Nasyam is also said to strengthen the mind and intellect and is included in pancha karma treatment.

PANCHA KARMA

The most famous form of Ayurvedic treatment is pancha karma. Pancha karma, or literally "five actions" in Sanskrit, is a cleansing treatment to increase the metabolic process with an appropriate diet, natural herbs, and minerals. Pancha karma is used for deep-rooted chronic diseases and seasonal imbalances of the three elemental energies (doshas): pitta, vata, and kapha. The treatment aims to make the body healthy by eliminating bodily waste products and achieving a balance between the doshas.

Pancha karma – five actions in three steps.

The five measures consist of nasyan (nasal treatment), vamana (vomiting), virechana (detoxing), nirooha vasti (enemas with herbal decoctions), and sneha vasti (enemas with herbal oils). After these treatments, hopefully, the body has been cleansed of accumulated toxins.

Panchakarma is always performed in three stages: purva karma (pre-treatment), pradhana karma (primary treatment) and paschat karma (post-treatment). The patient who chooses any of the five treatments above must always undergo all three stages for the treatment to have the intended effect.

Step 1. Pre-treatment (purva karma).
Snehana (oil therapy) is an essential preparatory treatment. Snehana is said to loosen toxins stuck in different places in the body and is often given with adapted herbal mixtures to treat an individual disease. Still, it can also be provided in a pure form without additives. Snehana is given early in the morning for a maximum of seven days and is said to help transfer toxins to the gastrointestinal tract so that they can be easily removed afterward. If snehana is not given before pancha karma, the intended effect on the treatment will not be obtained.

Oil massage (abhyanga) is another crucial treatment in pancha karma.

Svedana is a therapy that induces sweating and is administered to the whole body or parts of the body, depending on the disease. Steam with added medicinal herbs is usually used, but it can also be achieved by having the patient sit under the sun while thirsty and hungry, covering their body with thick sheets, or staying in a closed, dark room. Svedana is said to dilate ducts in the body and thus helps move toxins to the gastrointestinal tract.

Step 2. Primary treatment (pradhana karma).
The toxins and slag products that reach the gastrointestinal tract are believed to be eliminated during the primary treatment.

One of the five primary treatments, vamana karma, is used for kapha diseases such as bronchitis, colds, coughs, asthma, sinusitis, and excess mucus. One to three days before vamana karma, one is treated with oil internally and externally through abhyanga (Ayurvedic massage) and internally with ghee (shredded butter) in the diet.

Step 3. Post-treatment (paschat karma).
The finishing treatment consists of adapted diets, appropriate physical effort, and intake of herbs to promote long-term health.

AYURVEDA AND SESAME OIL
Sesame oil is extracted from sesame seeds and is often used in cooking as a seasoning, but in Ayurveda, it is also used for massage and skin care. It has been used for thousands of years in India due to its healing effects.

In Ayurveda, regular massage with sesame oil is recommended to achieve many health benefits. Ayurveda practitioners believe that massage with sesame oil cleanses, balances the lymphatic and endocrine systems, lubricates, and softens muscles, tissues, and joints. They also think that the oil makes the skin radiant and youthful. Sesame oil is the best oil to use due to its ability to penetrate the skin and because it is generally recommended for all body constitutions, whether you are a vata, kapha, or pitta.

According to Ayurveda, sesame oil is excellent because it is naturally antibacterial against common skin pathogens, such as staphylococci and streptococci, and common skin fungi, such as athlete's foot. It is also naturally antiviral and anti-inflammatory.

Additionally, sesame oil is considered to relieve or cure psoriasis, dry scalp, irritated skin, and skin rashes in teens, regulate pore enlargement, and heal or protect wounds.

AYURVEDIC MASSAGE IN THE HOME
How to do Ayurvedic oil massage at home.

1. Before starting the massage, warm the oil to body temperature or higher. Start by massaging your head. Dip your fingertips into the oil and massage the oil into the scalp. During the entire massage, use as much of the whole palm of your hand as possible, not just the fingertips. Since the head is one of the most essential body parts to massage, feel free to spend more time there than the other parts.

2. Gently lubricate the face and outer ears—massage with the entire palm where possible. Massage your face and neck gently. Do not massage as firmly here as on other body parts.

3. Then massage the neck and upper spine with open hands and light movements.

4. It is good to apply the oil on all body parts and then start again from the top and massage. This way, the oil has time to stay on the skin longer.

5. *Continue with your arms. Massage with reciprocating movements (long up and down movements) along the long muscles and circulating movements over the joints.*

6. *Proceed to the chest and abdomen—massage over the heart with light circular motions. Massage the abdomen clockwise from the lower right side upwards to the more down left side.*

7. *Massage all parts of the back and spine as far as you can.*

8. *Continue with the legs—massage with reciprocating movements along the large muscles and circulating movements over the joints.*

9. *Finally, massage your feet. Like the head, the feet are considered one of the most essential body parts to rub. Please spend a little more time here. Massage the soles of the feet with the entire palm.*

10. *Finish with a hot bath or shower.*

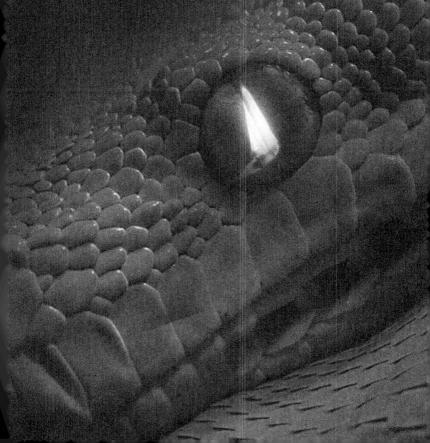

ESOTERIC
YOGA

Learn the hidden secrets,
Maithuna & Sexmagic!

ESOTERIC YOGA

THE WAY OF HIDDEN KNOWLEDGE

Esoteric means "inaccessible" or "only for the initiated" and is most often used to denote the hidden wisdom or secret spiritual knowledge that underlies philosophical systems. The term esoteric can also refer to the teachings and practices of supersensible experiences that require special preparation and training, often under the guidance of an experienced teacher.

One might wonder why knowledge is hidden. The answer is multifaceted, but in addition to the fact that the mysterious and hidden have an appeal to new students, it has a purely practical explanation. For example, if someone is only temporarily curious, they will most likely forget a mantra told to them, even if it could be life-saving. Tradition – the knowledge of it – will go nowhere. On the other hand, if a person undergoes demanding yogic and tantric training for years, that person will be more likely to remember the mantra. Keeping the knowledge hidden ensures that it is passed on and preserved for the future.

According to an old prophecy, the hidden, esoteric, tantric acts would one day be practiced quite openly – during Kali's age – which is now. It allows me to write about the most advanced tantric rituals previously hidden. However, I can not reveal everything. I can not tell you everything about things that can be abused. For example, I will not show the most potent mantra there is, the Shodasi mantra. A mantra that can replace all other secret mantras and gives the holder the power to influence everything in the macro and microcosm: the power of life and death, success and defeat. However, I can tell you about other previously hidden ones, the rituals that are refined through training and give the adept an increased awareness and vitality to successfully deal with everything in life. There is no point in not telling about that knowledge, in not passing it on. It would be like not telling interested people where they can find the best running shoes. Everything that can make it easier for people to have increased vitality and joy in life must now be acknowledged. The time has come. The time is now. The time is yours. Good luck!

THE PATH OF THE RIGHT AND LEFT HANDS

In tantra, the basis of all yoga, the hidden knowledge is preserved in two directions or paths: the path of the right hand (dakshinachara) and the path of the left hand (vamachara). Both paths aim to awaken Kundalini Shakti and give the practitioner cosmic power. Both paths are considered equal ways of enlightening the Indian tantric practitioners, although vamachara is regarded as the faster and more dangerous way.

DAKSHINACHARA

Dakshinachara is also described as the inner way or the path of meditation. Rituals are based on the practitioner's inner meditation, such as Kriya yoga.

VAMACHARA

Vamachara, the path of external meditation, is often the path that people know in tantra, where the adept gets help from things and experiences in the outside world to expand power—for example, the use of meat and wine in the maithuna ritual (tantric intercourse).

Both paths use secret mantras and yantras in their tantric rituals to achieve their purposes.

MANTRA SHASTRA

Mantra shastra is the foundation of all spiritual practice and is central to all esoteric yoga.

MANTRA
The most basic mantra is Aum, also known as the pranava mantra, the source of all mantras.

Two types of mantras which have a literal meaning are:

1.) SAGUNA MANTRA
Mantras that represent and invoke a deity, God, or goddess for spiritual self-realization. Saguna mantras create visual patterns through repeated chanting until the deity appears appropriately.

Some examples of saguna mantras are:

a) Om Namah Shivaya. Greetings to Shiva.
b) Om Nam Narayanaya. Greetings to God over harmony and balance.
c) Gayatri mantra. Dedicated to the goddess Gayatri.
d) Mahamrityunjaya mantra. Dedicated to Shiva.

More similar mantras are shanti mantra, Ram, Sita, Om Aing Saraswati Namaha, etc.

2.) NIRGUNA MANTRA
Mantras that are formless, abstract, and represent the universe as a whole and not in any specific form are called nirguna mantras. These

mantras require a higher form of concentration as they do not refer to any actual form. They are for more profound meditation, and with regular practice, siddhis (paranormal abilities) are obtained. The use of nirguna mantras is primarily to become one with the absolute or to identify with the divine in the universe. Some examples of nirguna mantras are:

a) Om (Aum). Om is the original mantra, the root of all sounds and letters that create language and thoughts.
b) So Ham. We unconsciously utter this mantra every time we breathe. On inhalation – So, and on exhalation – Ham. So Ham means – I am that, beyond the limitations of the mind and body, I am one with the infinite. I am. That's me.

There are primarily ten different types of magic mantras without a literal meaning:

1. Shanti (Siddhi) mantra – to free oneself from disease, fear, imagination, and other problems.

2. Stambhan's mantra is to make living beings unable to move.

3. Mohana mantra – used to create attraction.

4. The Uchchatan mantra is used to create mental imbalances in people.

5. Vashikaran mantra – used to turn someone into an enslaved person.

6. The Akarshan mantra is used to acquire wealth and material happiness.

7. The Jrambhan mantra is used to change human behavior.

8. The Vidweshan mantra is used to make two people enemies.

9. Maran mantra – used to kill someone.

10. The Paustik mantra is used to become successful on all levels.

SRI VIDYA MANTRA – SHODASI MANTRA

Sri Yantra – also known as Sri Chakra – is the mother of all yantras because all others are descended from it. It is the most potent yantra and symbolizes the creation of the cosmos and all life. Sri Vidya is worshiped by the tantric of both the right and left hands.

Sri Vidya or Sri Chakra represents Sri Lalita or Tripura Sundari – Shakti in her most beautiful form, a sixteen-year-old beauty. Sixteen syllables represent Sri Lalita as she is also associated with sixteen desires.

Since Sri Yantra is the most potent yantra, it also possesses the most powerful mantra – the Shodasi mantra. It is logical if you think about it, as each form also has a sound.

The Shodasi mantra is the most secret and protected and is impossible to find out about – unless a guru initiates you. Forget all the internet pages claiming to know the mantra because it is entirely wrong and unreasonable. If you have undergone all the trials that it means to be initiated, you do not give it away – especially not on the internet.

SRI YANTRA

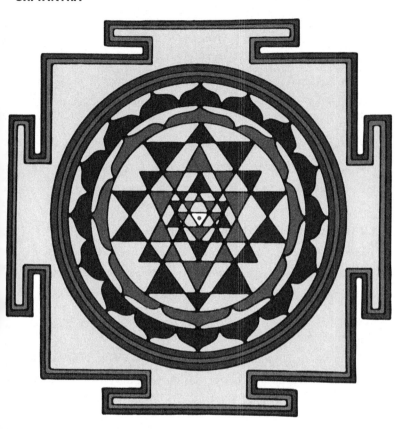

 Anahata Chakra

Manipura Chakra

Swadisthana Chakra

Moladhara Chakra

• Bindu

▽ Guru Chakra

 Soma Chakra

 Ajna Chakra

 Vishuddhi Chakra

319

Typically, one does not initiate the Shodasi mantra directly; the guru decides which time and place is most favorable. Generally, you are first started in the Bala mantra, then depending on your maturity and insight, you are initiated in the Panchadasi mantra. The Panchadasi mantra is a mantra made up of fifteen stages syllables. If the guru thinks the adept is ready for final liberation, he is initiated into the Shodasi mantra and gains knowledge of the secret sixteenth stage.

For the adept to achieve complete liberation and obtain magical abilities, so-called siddhis, he must recite the mantra nine hundred thousand times and add purascharana each time at the end.

BRAHMA VIDYA – THE BIGGEST SECRET
Shodashi vidya is also called Brahma vidya: Brahman (the world soul) and Vidya (the knowledge). Brahman is rendered into mantra form in Shodasi vidya, and because of this, it is guarded as the greatest secret.

Suppose the practitioner can reach the fourth level of consciousness, turiya (superconsciousness). In that case, he is most likely prepared to go beyond this to get the fifth level of consciousness, turiyatita. Turiyatita can be achieved without difficulty when the Shodasi mantra is recited regularly.

Therefore, you become one with Brahman by reaching turiyatita (the fifth level of consciousness) and reciting the Shodasi mantra. There is nothing after this.

What happens when a person is transformed into turiyatita? The world soul, the divine consciousness, replaces the soul. You become divine and gain divine power.

It is also something that can be experienced in a moment of near death; a person is never the same after such an experience.

BIJA MANTRA

Mantras often used in tantra are bija mantras. They are different sounds that have no direct literal meaning, but that has the power to create a significant transformation and expansion of the physical, emotional, and mental forces. They are called bija mantras, or so-called magical sounds.

The approximately fifty sacred sounds from the Sanskrit alphabet (bija mantras) are primarily resonants for the seven major chakras. Correctly stated, they activate the energy in different chakras and purify and balance the mind and body. They also increase the power of various mantra compositions.

AIM

After Om (Aum), the second most common bija mantra is Aim, pronounced – Aym. The Aim is the feminine aspect of Om and often follows Om in various mantras. Om and Aim consist of two compound vowels, including all sounds.

Om helps to purify the mind, and Aim helps to focus in different ways.

Just as Om is the sound of the invisible, Aim is the sound of the visible. Om is the sound of the unmanifested, and Aim is the sound of the manifested. The principle of consciousness and energy. Shiva and Shakti. Therefore, one can often hear Aim in Shakti mantras. Mantras of the Divine Mother. The Aim is the bija mantra for Saraswati, the goddess of knowledge and speech. Aim helps us in education, art, expression, and communication and is suitable for all forms of school work in general. The Aim is also a guru mantra and helps us to have more excellent knowledge of everything. It also helps us with concentration during the recitation of the mantras.

HRIM

After Om and Aim, Hrim pronounced "Hreem," the most common bija mantra. It combines the sound Ha, which stands for energy / prana, space, and light, with the sound of Ra, which stands for fire, light, and learning, and the sound A, which stands for energy, concentration, and motivation.

Hrim is bija mantra for Shakti or Parvati.

Hrim is a mantra for magic, attraction, love, and power. It brings us joy, ecstasy, passion, and complete happiness.

Hrim is a specific mantra for the heart (hridaya in Sanskrit) on all its levels: spiritually, emotionally, as a chakra, and as a physical organ.

SRIM

Srim, pronounced "Shreem," is one of the most common bija mantras due to its favorable properties. It attracts everything that is good and favorable and helps us develop positively.

Srim is the bija mantra of Lakshmi and is also called the Ramas bija when used to worship Lord Rama.

Srim is the mantra of faith, devotion, refuge, and surrender. It can be used to take shelter in or indulge in various deities and obtain their favors.

Srim relates to the heart more from a feminine and sentimental perspective, while Hrim relates to the heart from a masculine, pranic, or functional perspective.

Srim is often used with Hrim as Hrim relates to the sun, and Srim relates to the moon.

KRIM

Krim is pronounced "Kreem," the most crucial bija mantra that begins with a harsh consonant. Krim begins with Ka, the first consonant in Sanskrit, which shows manifested prana and the initial energy phase. To Ka, it adds the Ra sound of fire and the A sound that concentrates power like the other Shakti mantras. Krim creates light just like Hrim and Srim but on a more specific and actualized level.

Krim is the bija mantra of Kali, the goddess of time, destruction, and transformation. Kali also creates the highest energy level within us.

Krim is the mantra of work, yoga, and the energy of transformation. It is known to be a bija mantra for yoga practitioners and is applied to awaken Kundalini Shakti within us. Krim stimulates higher perceptiveness and prana and stabilizes pratyahara within us. The mantra can create contact with any deity.

KLIM

Klim is pronounced "Kleem" and is the softer, more feminine aspect of Krim. Just as Krim is electric, Klim is magnetic and attracts things to us.

*Klim relates to Akarshana Shakti or the law of attraction. Klim is
the bija mantra for Krishna and Sundari, the goddesses of love and
beauty. It is also the bija mantra over all desires (kama bija) and helps
us achieve our inner desires. Klim is the mantra of love and devotion
and increases the level of love within us. Because of this, it is one of the
most used mantras.*

STRIM

*Strim, pronounced "Streem," is composed of the Sa sound, which stands
for stability, and the Ta sound, which creates expansion, with the A
sound, which provides us with energy, direction, and motivation.*

*Strim is known to be the peace mantra, the so-called shanti bija. The
mantra Strim provides the power to have children, enrich something
nutritionally, protect, and guide. It is similar to Srim but more robust
and has a more stabilizing effect.*

*Strim is the bija mantra of the Hindu goddess Tara (not the Buddhist
Tara). Hindu Tara is associated with Durga, often called Durga-Tara,
a guarding and protective form of the goddess.*

HUM

*Hum is pronounced "Hoom" and is one of the most essential bija
mantras, along with Om, Aim, and Hrim. It is said to be Pranava, the
sound of Lord Shiva.*

*Hum is the great agni or fire mantra and can increase the fire within
us at all levels—everything from the fire of consciousness to the pranic
fire to the burning of the body.*

Hum is also a weapon, a protecting mantra that can destroy negativity with its enlightening fire. It is also called the bija mantra of anger (krodha bija).

Hum relates to a violent form of the goddess, like Kali, Chandi or Chinnamasta.

Hum raises Kundalini Shakti with breathing and concentration on the navel (Manipura chakra).

THE SECRET CHAKRAS

In yoga, people usually talk about seven or eight more significant chakras along the spine and at the top of the head. If you count Bindu visarga as a chakra, you say that a human has eight major vital chakras. According to popular belief, Bindu is located on the top of the back of the head and has no kshetram.

In the hidden tradition, you learn a big secret: Bindu's placement on the back of the head is the chakra's kshetram. That Bindu is located above the Sahasrara chakra and is called Sunya. When the Kundalini Shakti reaches the Sunya – the black chakra, one is transformed into a deity and receives divine qualities.

In addition to Sunya, other chakras are hidden: Guru, Nirvana, Indu, Manas, and Tala (Lalana) chakras are placed in the head, and Hrit chakra is placed just below the Anahata chakra, the heart chakra.

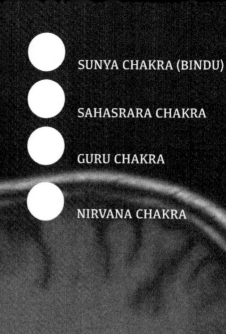

SUNYA CHAKRA (BINDU)

SAHASRARA CHAKRA

GURU CHAKRA

NIRVANA CHAKRA

INDU CHAKRA

MANAS CHAKRA

AJNA CHAKRA

TALU CHAKRA

THE HIDDEN RITUALS

KRIYA YOGA

There are seventy-two kriyas, of which twenty are the most used and suitable for daily use by any student. These kriyas are divided into three groups:

1. *Those who evoke pratyahara.*
2. *Those who evoke dharana.*
3. *Those that induce dhyana.*

KRIYAS FOR PRATYAHARA:

VIPAREETA KARANI MUDRA

Come into vipareeta karani asana. Ensure the legs are straight and the chin does not touch the chest. Close your eyes and breathe ujjayi pranayama. Experience in an inhalation how the amrit or nectar flows along the spine from the Manipura to the Vishuddhi chakra and gathers there. Hold your breath for a while and experience how the nectar gets cool. Then, exhale with ujjayi breathing and experience how the nectar flows from Vishuddhi through Ajna, Bindu, and Sahasrara. After exhaling, take the consciousness to Manipura again and repeat the kriya twenty-one times.

CHAKRA ANUSANDHANA

Sit in a meditation position and close your eyes. Breathe normally. Take consciousness to the Mooladhara chakra and follow the front passage "arohan" up to the Bindu. Repeat all the chakras up, Mooladhara, Swadhisthana, Manipura, Anahata, and Vishuddhi, and go from here directly to Bindu. Then, let the consciousness go down along the back passage and repeat the chakras on the way down. You are starting from Ajna, Vishuddhi, Anahata, Manipura, Swadhisthana, and Mooladhara. Then, start immediately on the next round, beginning with Swadhisthana. Please do not overdo it by trying to locate the chakras, but flow past them quickly. Practice nine rounds.

NADA SANCHALANA

Sit in a meditation position. Exhale completely. Open your eyes and bend your head down without pressing your chin against your chest. Take consciousness to the Mooladhara chakra. Silently repeat, "Mooladhara, Mooladhara, Mooladhara." Inhale and let the consciousness flow through the anterior passage "arohan" up to Bindu. Repeat the names of the chakras on the way up. When passing from Vishuddhi to Bindu, tilt your head slightly backward. Hold your breath and silently say "Bindu, Bindu, Bindu" to yourself. Then, continue down the back passage "awarohan" while saying the mantra Om inwardly. Close your eyes as you go down and experience the chakras. When you arrive at Mooladhara, hold your breath and repeat "Mooladhara" three times. Then, continue directly to the next round. Practice thirteen rounds.

PAWAN SANCHALANA

Sit in a meditation position and close your eyes. Practice khechari mudra and ujjayi pranayama. Exhale entirely and tilt your head down as in the previous kriya. Become aware of the Mooladhara chakra and silently repeat, "Mooladhara, Mooladhara, Mooladhara." Then inwardly say "arohan" and inhale with ujjayi breathing along the front passage while experiencing the chakras and mentally repeating their names. When you pass from Vishuddhi to Bindu, tilt your head back and silently repeat "Bindu, Bindu, Bindu." Then inwardly say "awarohan" and exhale along the back passage with ujjayi breathing. Repeat

the name of the chakras silently and close your eyes slowly as you move
down. Then open your eyes, tilt your head down, and start the next
round. Practice forty-nine rounds.

SHABA SANCHALANA

Sit in a meditation position. Practice khechari mudra and ujjayi pra-
nayama. Exhale entirely and open your eyes. Bend your head forward
and pay attention to the Mooladhara chakra briefly. Inhale with ujjayi
breathing and ascend along the anterior passage. Experience what
the sound of breathing So sounds like on the way up. Experience each
kshetram at the same time without any mental repetition. Tilt your
head back at the transition from Vishuddhi to Bindu. Hold your breath
and experience Bindu for a few seconds. Exhale, close your eyes, and
hear the sound of the breath, Ham. Experience each chakra on the way
down without rehearsing mentally. When you get to Mooladhara, open
your eyes, bend your head, and start the next round. Practice fifty-nine
rounds.

MAHA MUDRA

Sit in siddhasana or siddha yoni asana with your heel pressed aga-
inst the Mooladhara. Practice khechari mudra, exhale entirely, and
tilt your head forward. Keep your eyes open at first. Silently repeat,
"Mooladhara, Mooladhara, Mooladhara." Climb upwards along the
"arohan" with an ujjayi inhalation. Experience each kshetram on the
way up. Raise your head as you pass from Vishuddhi to Bindu. At Bin-
du, repeat "Bindu, Bindu, Bindu" internally. Practice moola bandha
and shambhavi mudra while holding your breath. Repeat mentally
"shambhavi, kechari, mool". When you say "shambhavi", focus on
the eyebrow center. When you say "kechari," focus on the tongue and
palate. When you say "mool," focus on the Mooladhara chakra. Repeat

this procedure thrice; accustomed practitioners repeat it twelve times—the first releases the shambhavi mudra and the moola bandha. Become aware of Bindu and walk down the back passage with ujjayi breathing to the Mooladhara chakra. Experience each chakra on the way down. With Mooladhara, tilt your head forward and open your eyes. Repeat "Mooladhara, Mooladhara, Mooladhara" and continue to the next round. Practice twelve rounds and finish with "Mooladhara, Mooladhara, Mooladhara".

MAHA BHEDA MUDRA

Sit as in the previous exercise. Practice khechari mudra and exhale completely. Keep your eyes open. Mentally repeat "Mooladhara, Mooladhara, Mooladhara." Inhale with ujjayi and ascend along the anterior passage to Bindu. As you pass from Vishuddhi to Bindu, lift your head. Repeat mentally, "Bindu, Bindu, Bindu." Go down the back passage to the Mooladhara with ujjayi breathing and close your eyes. Experience the chakras on the way down. Then, practice the jalandhara bandha while holding your breath. Practice nasikagra drishti, uddiyana bandha, and moola bandha. Mentally repeat "nasikagra, uddiyana, mool" and experience its seats in the body. Repeat the procedure three times as a beginner and twelve times when you are more accustomed. Release nasikagra drishti, moola bandha, uddiyana bandha and jalandhara bandha. Hold your head down and experience Mooladhara. Repeat "Mooladhara, Mooladhara, Mooladhara" mentally. Continue to the next round. Practice twelve rounds.

MANDUKI MUDRA

Sit in bhadrasana. Keep your eyes open. The body surface under the Mooladhara should be in contact with the floor. Place a pillow or blanket under you if necessary. Place your hands on your knees and prac-

*tice nasikagra drishti. Become aware of the natural breath that flows
through your nostrils. On inhalation, respiration flows through both
nostrils and meets at the center of the eyebrows. On exhalation, the
flow separates at the center of the eyebrows and through the nostrils—
experience how breathing follows a V-shaped pattern. Be aware of all
odors. The point of the kriya is to share the smell of the astral body,
which is the smell of sandalwood. If your eyes get tired, close them for
a while. Do the exercise until it feels intoxicating. Please do not get
caught in it, but quit before you are absorbed by it too much.*

TADAN KRIYA

*Sit in padmasana with your eyes open. Place your hands next to your
body on the floor with your fingers pointing forward. Tilt your head
back and practice shambhavi mudra. Inhale through the mouth with
ujjayi breathing. When you inhale, experience how the breathing sinks
downwards through a tube between the mouth and the Mooladhara
chakra. Hold your breath, experience the Mooladhara chakra, and
practice the moola bandha. Using your hands, lift your body off the
floor and lower it so the Mooladhara lightly hits the floor. Repeat three
to eleven times. Then, exhale through the nose with ujjayi breathing.
Practice seven times.*

KRIYAS FOR DHARANA:

NAUMUKI MUDRA

*Sit in a meditation position. Keep your eyes closed throughout the
exercise. Make sure to have pressure at Mooladhara; use a pillow or
blanket if necessary.*

Make the khechari mudra and bend your head gently downwards.

Mentally repeat "Mooladhara, Mooladhara, Mooladhara." Inhale through the anterior passage to the Bindu. Raise your head as you pass from Vishuddhi to Bindu. Practice shanmuki mudra. Block the ears with the thumbs, the eyes with the index fingers, the nostrils with the middle fingers, the upper lip with the ring fingers, and the lower lip with the little fingers—practice moola bandha and varjoli / sahajoli mudra. Experience the passage along the spine to Bindu. Visualize a trident in copper at the bottom of the Mooladhara. The shaft runs along the spine, and the prongs point upwards from Vishuddhi. The trident rises spontaneously several times, and its middle prong pierces Bindu. When it penetrates Bindu, you mentally say "Bindu bhedan". After a while, release the varjoli / sahajoli mudra and moola bandha and drop your hands on your knees—Exhale from the Bindu with ujjayi breathing along the posterior passage and down to the Mooladhara. Say "Mooladhara, Mooladhara, Mooladhara," mentally. Repeat the exercise. Practice five rounds and finish by exhaling.

SHAKTI CHALINI

Sit in a meditation position. Keep your eyes closed throughout the exercise. Practice khechari mudra. Exhale completely, tilt your head forward, and experience Mooladhara. Repeat mentally, "Mooladhara, Mooladhara, Mooladhara," and then ascend along the front passage to Bindu with ujjayi breathing. Lift your head when you reach Bindu. Hold your breath and practice shanmukhi mudra. Let the consciousness flow continuously down the back passage and up along the front passage while holding your breath. Visualize a narrow green snake moving along the psychic passage. Its head is at Bindu, and it bites its tail. When you follow the snake, you can see how it starts to move along the passage or even make its passages. Look at the snake, no matter what it does. When you need to exhale, release your hands and *experience Bindu. Go down the back passage with ujjayi pranayama. Repeat "Mooladhara, Mooladhara, Mooladhara," and ascend along the front passage. Practice five times without interruption.*

SHAMBHAVI

Sit in a meditation position. Close your eyes and practice khechari mudra. Visualize a lotus flower with a long green stalk extending downwards. The roots are white or transparent green. The roots spread outwards from the Mooladhara chakra. The lotus flower is at the Sahasrara chakra and is closed like a bud. At the bottom of the bud are some light green leaves. The fallen petals of the flower are pink with delicate red veins. Try to see the lotus. You visualize it in chidakasha and feel it all over your body. Exhale and take consciousness to the root of the Mooladhara chakra. Inhale with ujjayi breathing and let your consciousness rise along the stem upwards along the spine. At the end of inhalation, you reach the bud of the flower. Keep your attention on the Sahasrara and hold your breath. You are inside the lotus flower but can also see it outside. It begins to unfold slowly. When the flower opens, you can see its yellow pollen sprinkled in the middle. The lotus closes and opens almost immediately again. When the lotus has stopped opening and closing, exhale with ujjayi and go down the stem to the Mooladhara. Stay there and experience how the roots spread in different directions. Repeat the exercise eleven times.

AMRIT PAN

Sit in a meditation position. Keep one eye closed and practice khechari mudra. Take consciousness to the Manipura chakra. A warm, sweet liquid is stored there. Exhale completely with ujjayi while taking a quantity of fluid to the Vishuddhi chakra along the spine. Stay at Vishuddhi for a while. The liquid that you brought with you from

Manipura is now cooled down. With ujjayi breathing, you exhale up to the Lalana chakra. Inflate the cold fluid up to the Lalana chakra using the breath. Take consciousness to the Manipura chakra again. Repeat the exercise nine times.

CHAKRA BHEDAN

Sit in a meditation position. Keep your eyes closed throughout the exercise. Practice khechari mudra and ujjayi pranayama. Breathe without interruption between inhaling and exhaling. Exhale and take consciousness to the Swadhisthana chakra. Inhale, bring consciousness to the Mooladhara chakra and up along the anterior passage. At Vishuddhi kshetram, breathing will end, and you will start exhaling immediately. Exhale from Vishuddhi kshetram to Bindu and then down the spine from Ajna to Swadhisthana chakra. It is a complete round. Practice fifty-nine rounds. If you become too introverted, finish the exercise and move on to the next kriya.

SUSHUMNA DARSHAN

Sit in a meditation position, close your eyes, and breathe normally. Take consciousness to the Mooladhara chakra. Imagine a pencil with which you draw a square at the Mooladhara chakra. Draw an inverted triangle inside the square. Then, make a circle that touches each corner of the square. Make four petals on each side of the square. Take consciousness to Swadhisthana. Draw a circle there as big as the previous one. Draw six petals around the circle and a crescent moon inside it. Take consciousness to Manipura. Draw a circle and draw an inverted triangle inside it. In the middle of it, you draw a fireball.

Make ten petals around the circle. Take consciousness to the Anahata. Draw two triangles that lie on each other, one with the tip up and the other with the tip down. Draw a circle around these with twelve petals. Then, take consciousness to Vishuddhi. Draw a circle with a smaller circle inside, like a drop of nectar. Make sixteen petals around the circle. Take consciousness to the eye. Draw a circle with the sign Om inside. Draw two large petals around the circle, one on the right and one on the left. For Bindu, draw a crescent moon with a small circle above it. At Sahasrara, make a circle with a triangle with the tip facing up. There are a thousand petals around the circle. Try to see all the chakras in their respective places. It can be challenging to see everything at once, so start by visiting two at a time and adding a new one for each day.

PRANA AHUTI

Sit in a meditation position. Close your eyes and breathe normally. Experience a light pressure on the top of the head, the pressure of a divine hand. The hand provides the body and mind with prana flowing down from the Sahasrara along the spine. You may experience this as cold, heat, electricity, or a stream of liquid or wind. When the prana has reached the Mooladhara chakra, you go directly to the next kriya.

UTTHAN

Sit in a meditation position. Close your eyes and breathe normally. Take consciousness to the Mooladhara chakra. Try to visualize it as detailed as you can. See a black Shiva lingam. The bottom of the lingam is cut away, and a small red snake moves around it. The snake tries to entangle itself so it can rise along the sushumna. While it struggles to eliminate it, it makes an angry hissing sound. The tail is attached to the Shiva lingam, but the body and head rise along the spine and then come down again. You may experience this as the body contracts, followed by happiness and bliss. When this occurs, move on to the next kriya.

SWAROOPA DARSHAN

Sit in a meditation position and keep your eyes closed. Become aware of your physical body. Your body is entirely still. You are as solid as a mountain. Become aware of your natural breathing while ensuring your body is completely still. Your body solidifies and becomes immobile. After a while, you are absorbed by the natural breath while your body thickens. When your body is so still that you cannot move it even though you want to, you move on to the next kriya.

LINGA SANCHALANA

Sit completely still with your eyes closed. Your breathing has automatically switched to ujjayi breathing, and you are practicing khechari mudra. Be fully aware of your breathing. With each inhalation, the body expands, and with each exhalation, it contracts. Your physical body is still entirely still; your astral body moves. After a while, you only experience the astral body. You may reach a stage where the astral body, during contraction, becomes a tiny point of light. When this happens, you go straight to the next kriya.

KRIYA FOR DHYANA:

DHYANA

You have experienced your astral body as a tiny point of light. Please look closer at the bright spot and how it resembles a golden egg. When you look at the egg, it begins to expand. It gets the same shape as your astral and physical body as it gets bigger. This form is neither material nor subtle; it is the form of pure light.

NOTE. This kriya for dhyana can be used as a conclusion in all yoga and all meditations, not only in Kriya yoga.

MAITHUNA

Maithuna, the tantric intercourse within the vamachara tradition, is perhaps the ritual most people associate with tantra. It is known as the most effective method for awakening our dormant, inner cosmic power – Kundalini Shakti. We awaken the Kundalini Shakti in the root chakra – Mooladhara chakra, and guide the energy up through the sushumna nadi along the spine, activating all our chakras. When it reaches the Sahasrara chakra, the crown chakra at the top of our head, we connect to the power of the cosmos and the collective consciousness. Our spine and chakras turn into an antenna that transmits but also receives. The longer we wait to release the orgasm, the stronger the signal becomes and the more power we are filled with. By practicing Maithuna regularly, we gradually become more enlightened.

Historically, the tantrikas of the vamachara tradition used the energy generated from sexual group rituals to obtain siddhis (paranormal / magical powers) and enlightenment. Every woman who participated became a goddess and every man a god. So it was not necessary, exactly, which counterpart one had in the sexual group activity. It was the spiritual experience that mattered and was at the center.

PREPARATION

Everything preceding the act is apt to raise awareness and remove tensions.

1. The room where the ritual occurs is clean; incense should be burned there. The nose and the olfactory organs are connected by nerves and acceptable psychic currents to the Mooladhara chakra, where the Kundalini is twisted. Your attention and sensitivity increase when the sense of smell is affected correctly.

2. Prepare food and flowers to be used during the ritual. The meal consists of four parts, and the room is decorated with flowers.

Pancha makara, tattwa chakra or pancha tattwa is also the name of the five "m" used in the ritual.

Wine – madya.

Wine symbolizes the intoxicating experience of the richness of consciousness achieved through yoga. If you prefer not to use alcohol, you can replace it with non-alcoholic wine or coconut milk. The element fire. Tattwa agni.

Meat – mamsa.

Flesh symbolizes "Everything I am, everything I do and experience – what I stand for, everything is part of my being." If you do not eat meat, replace it with garlic, ginger, sesame seeds, tofu, or other soy products. The element earth. Tattwa prithvi.

Fish – matsya.

Fish symbolizes a state where "I experience everything, the whole universe, pleasure, and pain, as myself. I am all this. I contain all opposites". If you do not eat fish, replace it with aubergines and radishes. The element water. Tattwa apas.

Roasted barley products – mudra.

Rice, wheat, etc. They symbolize that "I stop identifying with fears and inhibitions." The element air. Tattwa vayu.

Flowers (represents intercourse) – maithuna.

Flowers symbolize intercourse, representing the original power, the feminine that rises to the highest chakra and unites with the masculine. The element space. Tattwa akasha.

3. Shower together. It is relaxing, invigorating, and prepares you both to meet your "divine partner." Shakti (the woman who symbolizes all women) is lubricated with fragrant oils and perfumes. Different oils can be rubbed into other body parts, such as musk oil around the Venus mountain.

Then, you especially massage your partner's spine. Start at the lower part of the spine, press your thumbs alternately with small movements back and forth, and work your way up along the spine. The area where the sushumna, ida, and pingala nadi flow is then released from tension and activated.

TO OPEN UP

The room has been decorated with flowers, the food has been served, and the wine has been poured; incense glows, candles are burning, or even better, an oil lamp that emits a red glow.

The next step in this holy experience is to inaugurate and cleanse the room and the house by sprinkling water and saying a mantra. A mantra with long lines of verse is usually used.

This part of the ritual is extensive and precisely laid out to keep the mind occupied. The mind comes in an elevated and secure state. Here, you can use the mantra – Aim Hrim Krom Hamsah So-Ham, repeated

aloud eleven times. To the house or surroundings, to the room, to those
present, to the food, to the wine, to the four directions, up and down.
The different bija mantras are often translated as other manifestations
of energy and consciousness. In this context, however, the mantra
represents "conscious attention."

Have a small bowl of water in front of you, dip your fingers in it,
sprinkle the water as above, and say the mantra Swaha (I burn it, I
donate it) each time. Also, dip some flowers in the water and throw
them on the food – Swaha, on the wine – Swaha, on those present –
Swaha ...

This act should last so long and thorough that you become wholly
preoccupied with it and can indulge in it seriously and without reser-
vation.

With his finger dipped in red powder mixed with a bit of soapy water
and oil, Shakti puts a red dot in the center of the eyebrows of those
present. She also gets a point. It symbolizes the ability for concentra-
tion and empathy achieved through the Ajna chakra in the middle of
the head. If Ajna's chakra is aroused, you will participate in this act
without tension, without being hampered by shame or frivolity.

YOGA AND MEDITATION

Do pranayamas and bandhas and yoga nidra. Then, use the So-Ham
(or your mantra) with ujjayi pranayama. Meditate with So-Ham – So
as you inhale, and Ham as you exhale. So-Ham means, "I am that – I
am part of the divine, I am God." Meditate on your body. Experience
your natural breathing until you reach a deep and calm state, then
repeat the mental mantra Aim Hrim Krom Hamsah So-Ham. Expe

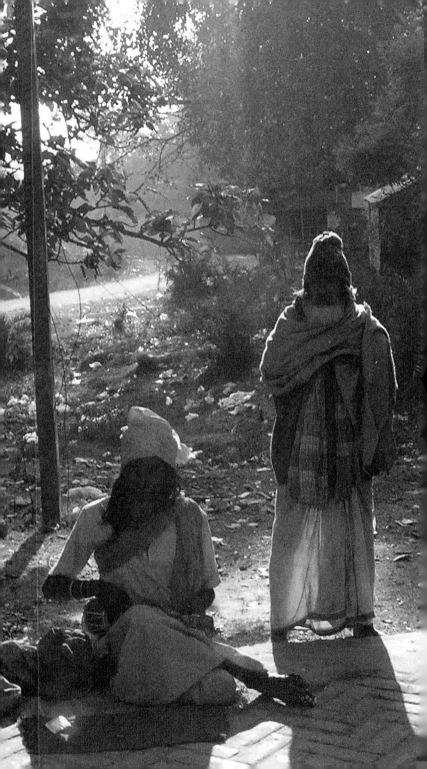

rience your body as light – imagine that the body is made of pure light and that this light destroys every fear in you, every inhibition, and all hatred. Experience that you are prepared for the cosmic act. You experience the union between the power – the feminine in you, and the consciousness – the masculine. Experience a strengthening and cleansing light flow that fills your body and breathing.

RITUALS

A guru is appointed to lead the ritual if several people are present. He dips his middle finger in the water and draws a downward-pointing triangle on the floor where you sit, and then over this, he draws an upward-pointing triangle. In the middle of both triangles – in the middle of the hexagonal star, draw a smaller square and, in the square, another downward-pointing triangle. A circle that touches all the corners is drawn around both triangles; then, eight petals are drawn around the outside of the circle.

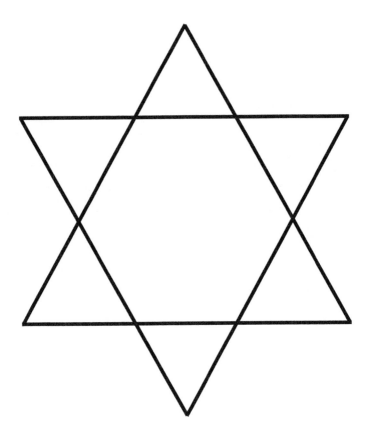

The two triangles symbolize the female and male parts of the universe.
Shiva and Shakti. Purusha and Prakriti. Consciousness and energy.

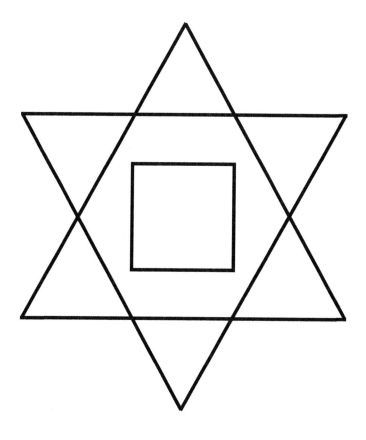

The square symbolizes the foundation from which the power is aroused and rises, the Mooladhara chakra.

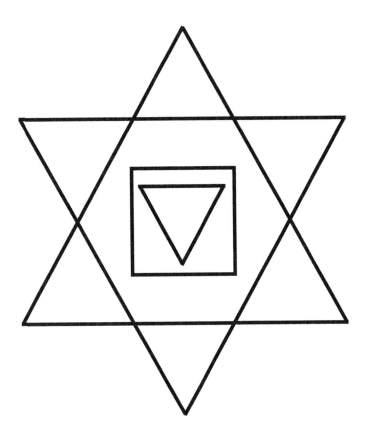

The force, Kundalini, is symbolized by the last triangle.

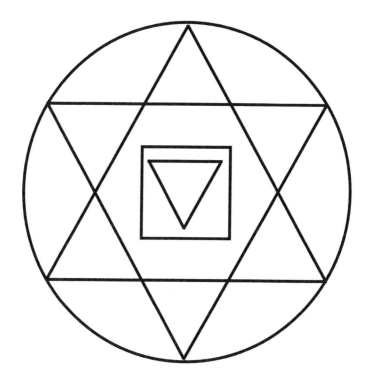

The circle symbolizes eternity.

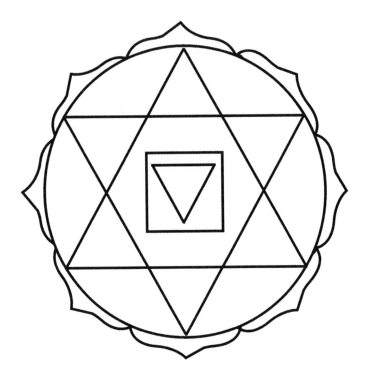

The petals symbolize infinity.

Finally, before the action itself, an essential part of the ritual comes: the wine is inaugurated by Shakti with flowers, water, and the mantra Swaha. She opens the wine to everyone present. The wine has a liberating effect on the mind, but do not drink too much. Consciousness must pass clearly.

The man sits in a meditation position. The woman sits on his left thigh. They give each other wine and food, feeding each other. If this position is too difficult, you can sit beside each other with the woman seated to the man's left.

Just as scents affect Mooladhara chakra, Swadhisthana chakra is affected by food and drink. All this increases the desire and sensitivity.

THE ACT

Sit opposite your partner – look each other in the eyes. You are entirely naked – two people, a man and a woman, and experience each other's sex and desire. You appreciate each other; two divine beings participate in a universal action.

Meditate on each other, and experience each other with desire and joy. If you smile from embarrassment or tense muscles in your face or body, return to the relaxed naturalness every time. Get back to the game and the seriousness of what you do repeatedly. If limiting thoughts arise – whatever happens, accept it and then return to the experience of each other.

Continue to experience your divine partner for a long time. You do not have to demand, explain, or excuse anything. You should not achieve anything – be, experience, enjoy!

The intercourse itself can be performed either in the following way or in one of the sixty-four tantric positions. In the tantric positions, you take a sexual yoga position. It is not done mechanically or by you getting up and sitting down again; it is done without losing touch with each other, even for a second. Remain immobile in every position …

POSITIONS

1. *The man sits in a meditation position, and the woman sits down on the man and wraps her legs around the man's waist and hips so that her feet are crossed behind his seat.*

2. *Same as 1 – but instead of the woman crossing her legs behind him, she lifts them while the man holds his arms under her knees and embraces her around the waist and lower back.*

3. *The man is lying on his back, and the woman is squatting on him.*

4. *The woman starts by sitting as in 3, then lies backward between the man's legs and stretches her legs along his body.*

5. *Standing. The man stands on the floor and holds the woman while she hangs on him with her legs and arms wrapped around him.*

6. *The woman lies stretched out on the man or vice versa. There are several variations; the back must be straight or in the yoga position. Remain immobile in the position while you experience each other mentally and physically. Together, you go into an uninterrupted sexual meditation. You are immobile. The experience of mental and physical union can come at any time, and when it comes, stay in it as long as it is at its peak, then end it.*

The shortest time in a position is more than half an hour to reach any fundamental transformation.

However, you do not have to worry about the body or the performance; let the Shakti in your partner lead you and your inspiration. Give and receive. Do not strive for a normal orgasm, but let the experience of each other transform you. The sixty-four positions symbolize freedom from expectations so you can do things differently each time. You decide for yourself.

Get used to the ritual; do it many times. Gradually, you will master it and get the full benefit of it. It will have a more profound effect when it can be done effortlessly.

In addition to the ritual performed by a couple, there are rituals shared by several couples sitting together in a circle. The introductory part of the ritual is performed by all couples together. The woman chosen to be Shakti for all present in the circle symbolizes power and is honored to be one. She pours the wine, leads the serving of the food, and thus begins the ritual. A guru performs the mantra ritual and guides the meditation and the process. During intercourse itself, in the different positions, each pair sits separately in a large circle called the chakra. The feast or ritual that raises consciousness is called puja – chakra puja.

Meditating with others creates a strong force field and supports everyone who participates. There are different puja: In the Bharai chakra, you have a partner appointed in advance. In yogini puja, you choose freely and independently of the individual.

A chakra puja can be done in different ways. Having intercourse as a ritual is so crucial that it can have a liberating effect on our lives. It becomes a beautiful and central act in human society.

SEX MAGIC

Sexual power and orgasm create life and are the most vital energy in the cosmos. Therefore, it is used in yoga, tantra, and magic to give the practitioner the ultimate power. It is logical and easy to understand.

After initiating sexual magic, you become a magician. The initiation takes place from man to woman and from woman to man. The guru – regardless of gender, passes on his magical powers to the adept via Shaktipat. The adept is initiated with the guru's orgasm.

Even if you do not possess the magical power of a magician, you can use your sexual magic rituals to get what you want, such as supernatural desire.

MAGICAL WISH

1. Write down / draw your wish on paper or use a picture of what you wish. Put it next to you and say the wish out loud to yourself.

2. Start masturbating and experience an inner image of desire in the Mooladhara chakra—experience how the image is in the chakra and turns dark red. Experience four petals that enclose the image.

3. Experience how you draw the image of the Swadhisthana chakra, how it turns orange, and how six petals enclose it.

4. Experience how you draw the image of the Manipura chakra, how it turns yellow, and how ten petals enclose it.

5. Experience how you draw the image to the Anahata chakra, how the picture turns blue, and how twelve petals enclose it.

6. Experience how you draw the image to the Vishuddhi chakra, how it becomes violet in color, and how sixteen petals enclose it.

7. Experience how you draw the image to the Ajna chakra, how the image turns white, and how the shape of a pyramid encloses it.

8. Experience how you draw the image to the Sahasrara chakra, how it turns purple-red, and how an infinite number of petals enclose it.

9. When the orgasm comes, you shoot the image out of the Sahasrara chakra, and you mentally experience how the desire leaves the scalp and goes away into the cosmos.

If you change after making your magical wish, you will burn up the image of the want so that it ceases to work.

Did you like the book? Feel free to follow me on my social media, share and like, tell your friends about the books, and feel free to write an honest review; one or two lines don't matter. All support is precious. Thanks!

On my Facebook page and Instagram, I post exciting news and tips on temporary offers and benefits you can take advantage of. I often also post my yoga routine and other things related to nutrition and health that may be interesting to take part in. So feel free to join them so you don't miss anything interesting:

 facebook.com/bhagwanoneofakindbooks

 instagram.com/bhagwanoneofakindbooks/

MY BOOKS AND BOOK SERIES

I have two book series that have different audiences. Great Yoga Books – is a series with the most comprehensive fact books on yoga for those who want to explore the subject in depth. Here, you will also find classic yoga books that are rarely translated, such as Patanjali's Yoga Sutras and Hatha Yoga Pradipika. My second series, Yoga Beyond the Poses: The Ultimate Beginner's Guide to Yoga, covers one yoga topic at a time and is extra easy to read with larger text. For those who find it challenging to read extensive books and want a good and broad overview of the subject quickly. Both series are also available as audiobooks.

★★★★★

TEACHING YOGA

&

MEDITATION

BEYOND

THE POSES

BESTSELLING AUTHOR

Shreyananda

Natha

Teaching Yoga and Meditation Beyond the Poses – A unique and practical workbook!

Teaching Yoga and Meditation Beyond the Poses – A unique and practical workbook for aspiring yoga teachers who want to teach yoga and meditation beyond the poses.

Teaching Yoga and Meditation Beyond the Poses is a unique and essential resource for new and experienced teachers and a guide for all yoga students interested in refining their skills and knowledge. Teaching Yoga and Meditation is also ideal as a core textbook in yoga teacher training programs.

The book covers fundamental yoga philosophy and history topics, including a historical presentation of classical yoga literature: Yoga Sutras of Patanjali, Bhagavad Gita, etc. Each of the seven major styles of yoga is described, from Hatha yoga, Raja yoga, Tantra yoga, Bhakti yoga, and Kundalini yoga, to knowledge about the chakras, Ayurveda and magic mantras and yantras. The book provides extensive support and tools for teaching integrated and classical yoga (asanas), breathing techniques (pranayamas), deep relaxation (Yoga Nidra), and meditation (Ajapa Japa). The book is divided into eight modules with associated knowledge tests and complete yoga and meditation classes.

https://rb.gy/9s6edj

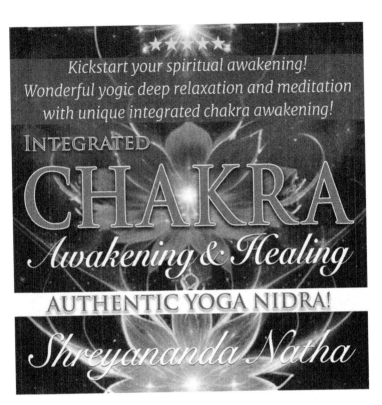

Printed in Great Britain
by Amazon